Normalizing Challenging or Complex Childbirth

Normalizing Challenging or Complex Childbirth

Edited by Karen Jackson and Helen Wightman

 Open University Press

Open University Press
McGraw-Hill Education
8th Floor
338 Euston Road
London
NW1 3BH

email: enquiries@openup.co.uk
world wide web: www.mheducation.co.uk

and Two Penn Plaza, New York, NY 10121-2289, USA

First published 2017

A catalogue record of this book is available from the British Library

ISBN-13: 978-0-33-526432-2
ISBN-10: 0-33-526432-8
eISBN: 978-0-33-526433-9

Library of Congress Cataloging-in-Publication Data
CIP data applied for

Typeset by Transforma Pvt. Ltd., Chennai, India

Fictitious names of companies, products, people, characters and/or data that may be used herein (in case studies or in examples) are not intended to represent any real individual, company, product or event.

Printed and bound by CPI Group (UK) Ltd, Croydon, CR0 4YY

Praise for this book

"Normalizing Challenging or Complex Childbirth, *edited by Karen Jackson and Helen Wightman, provides an insightful and informative perspective on an array of midwifery issues pertinent to today's society, including: obesity, VBAC and diabetes.*

Karen Jackson's first chapter 'The concept of normality in the context of challenging or complex childbirth' *sets the standard for additional eminent contributing authors; and they follow with an engaging exploration and explanation of the issues which is seamless in terms of application to practice and is supported by real life case studies and key practice points. This is a must read resource for midwives, students and educators."*

Janet Israel, *Midwifery Lecturer, Cardiff University, UK*

"Normalizing Challenging or Complex Childbirth *provides midwives and students with a refreshingly practical and sensitive approach to caring for women when pregnancy and birth bring additional physiological challenges. New and emerging evidence on important clinical scenarios is presented with great compassion in the context of contemporary midwifery care. This book will be an important resource to midwives wishing to provide individualized sensitive care to women facing the challenge of an unexpected, or complex, pregnancy path."*

Julia Sanders, *PhD Consultant Midwife and Reader in Midwifery, Cardiff University, UK*

I would like to dedicate this book to my lovely little family:
Gabriel and Megan, with all my love Karen (aka wife and Mum)

Helen and I would also like to dedicate this book to all
the childbearing women
and midwives out there. Your courage is an inspiration.

Contents

List of editors and contributors

Jenny Bailey, Assistant Professor in Midwifery, Division of Midwifery, University of Nottingham, UK.

Jane Evans, Independent Midwife at UKBC, Dorset, UK.

Dr. Clare Gribbin, Consultant in Obstetrics, Maternal Medicine and Psychosexual Medicine, Nottingham University Hospitals NHS Trust, UK.

Kathryn Gutteridge, Consultant Midwife and clinical lead for low-risk care, Sandwell and West Birmingham Hospitals NHS Trust, UK.

Karen Jackson, Assistant Professor in Midwifery and PhD student, Division of Midwifery, University of Nottingham, UK.

Angela Kerrigan, Consultant Midwife, Arrowe Park Hospital, Wirral University Teaching Hospital NHS Foundation Trust and PhD student (NMAHP Research Unit), University of Stirling, UK.

Professor Helen Spiby, Professor in Midwifery, School of Health Sciences, University of Nottingham, UK and Honorary Professor, School of Nursing and Midwifery, University of Queensland, Australia.

Mary Ellen Vance, Local Supervising Authority Midwifery Officer. North of Scotland LSA Consortium (hosted by NHS Highland). Retired July 2015.

Dr. Denis Walsh, Associate Professor in Midwifery, Division of Midwifery, University of Nottingham, UK.

Helen Wightman, Assistant Professor in Midwifery, Division of Midwifery, University of Nottingham, UK.

Foreword

For most of human history, the majority of pregnant and labouring women and babies have been assumed to be healthy, unless complications are actually present. However, as many researchers, policy-makers, and activists have noted, within a very short timespan (in terms of the whole of human history) a general fear of risk in societies around the world has led to highly risk-averse maternity systems. This has gradually shifted pregnant and labouring women from being seen as either 'healthy' or 'ill' to being 'low risk' (i.e., not yet ill, and in need of testing and screening) or 'high risk' (i.e., in need of treatment and interventions, just in case). This has the effect of narrowing the definition of 'normal' for women and babies with no identifiable clinical or psychological conditions, and of eliminating it altogether for those with such conditions. This book provides a welcome counterbalance. It turns the conversation of risk and abnormality around, by providing practical insights into ways of maximising the physiological potential of women and babies who might otherwise be classified as deviating from the 'norm', or as 'challenging' or 'high risk' and therefore without hope of experiencing as normal a pregnancy and birth as possible. In so doing, it offers a theoretical, and, importantly, clinical guide to how to maximise the physiological capacity of women with a wide range of challenging or potentially complicating conditions during pregnancy and labour. This is particularly timely in the context of an emerging turn in the global conversation towards the philosophy of midwifery (as practised by midwives and others) to improve outcomes and the lives of women, babies, and families. Ultimately, the book acts as a critique to current binary notions of low/high risk; ill/healthy; or normal/abnormal. It offers a vision of what maternity services might look like if they were truly focused on a philosophy of 'unique normality' for all, and not just for the few who are lucky enough to fit the increasingly narrow standards of being low risk. Vitally, it provides practical case studies, hints, and tips for making this change happen for each individual mother and baby, and, therefore, for all mothers and babies.

Soo Downe, Professor in Midwifery Studies,
School of Community Health and Midwifery,
University of Central Lancashire (UCLAN), UK
May 2016

Preface

This book was conceived as a result of both personal and professional experiences. In Chapter 1, one of us (Karen) describes her birth experience and how a really simple act made a world of difference to her and the midwife caring for her.

Both of us (Helen and Karen) teach on a module that covers complexity or challenges in childbirth, but we also teach on normality workshops. We therefore have a shared passion not only for promoting normality in childbirth but also for normalizing or humanizing childbirth regardless of 'risk' status.

It is well documented that complexity in childbirth is increasing, which is the result of a number of factors, including increasing maternal age, rising levels of obesity and related diabetes. We notice in our own clinical practice that when women are labelled as moderate or high risk, they immediately follow a pathway of increased surveillance and subsequent interventions that may or may not be clinically indicated. As a consequence, women are often excluded from qualitative strategies that so-called 'low-risk women' enjoy. Such approaches include water immersion for labour, aromatherapy and simply mobilization. In the antenatal period, high-risk women may only see obstetricians during clinic visits, depriving them of seeing a midwife to discuss very normal aspects of childbirth such as preparation for labour and birth or infant feeding choices.

Such strategies may be just as helpful – if not more so – for women with complex or challenging pregnancy as women with a straightforward pregnancy. Following a purely medicalized, technocratic model of childbirth can adversely affect the whole experience of childbirth, and lead to feelings of disempowerment and dissatisfaction.

This book was developed to assist and support midwives and student midwives in helping women from all risk categories to achieve the most optimum childbirth experience for their own unique circumstances. The text may also be useful for obstetricians and medical students who wish to provide more holistic maternity care. We acknowledge that many maternity units already employ many of the strategies suggested and provide an excellent service for all in their care. However, many other maternity units may have very different care pathways for different childbearing women depending on their risk status. The chapters contain many helpful hints and tips to help normalize or humanize childbirth, in particular the 'Practice points' and 'Reflection points'. And most of the chapters contain case studies based on women's or midwives' own real-life experiences (confidentiality is maintained where appropriate), which powerfully exemplify the significant affirmative impact of optimizing and normalizing childbirth.

Clearly, this book does not cover all the aspects of normalizing or humanizing childbirth. We would have liked to include chapters on maternal age, water immersion/birth, aromatherapy and other complementary therapies, to name a few, but restrictions of space prevented this. Maybe these will appear in another volume, or someone else might take up the mantle.

We are, however, delighted that in addition to the chapters we have written ourselves, there are contributions from some eminent midwives who have their own specialist interest or expertise. There is also a chapter by a consultant obstetrician who shares our philosophy of promoting optimum childbirth. She counsels women who have a profound fear of childbirth.

In light of the publicity surrounding the Kirkup Report in 2015 (see Chapter 2), it is absolutely vital that we make the point that we in no way imply that normalizing or humanizing childbirth should ever compromise the safety or well-being of childbearing women and their babies. We do believe that a positive, satisfying childbirth experience and a safe one are not mutually exclusive. Indeed, we and many midwives believe that the two are most definitely achievable.

Finally, we hope that this book challenges and prompts midwives and students of midwifery to evaluate their local services and provide them with the background tools and inspiration to make changes in their sphere of practice to improve the choices and outcomes for women.

1

The concept of normality in the context of challenging or complex childbirth

Karen Jackson

Introduction

In many cultures throughout history, birth has been viewed as a highly significant event, marked by particular rites and rituals that often have spiritual and cultural meanings (Kitzinger, 2000). Narratives around childbirth include descriptions of it being a profound, transformative and powerful human experience (Lavender et al., 2009). Women often recount 'feelings of empowerment, elation and achievement, although other women's experiences include trauma, fear, pain, and loss of control' (Lavender et al., 2009: 2). According to Kitzinger (2005), the change from women giving birth in a familiar home environment surrounded by female attendants, to women giving birth in an institutionalized setting surrounded by technology has contributed to this alternative discourse of trauma and fear. The net result of this change, according to some authors (Downe and McCourt, 2008; McCourt, 2010; Walsh, 2012), is a reduction in the occurrence and experience of birth without intervention.

This book explores challenging or complex childbirth and therefore it is acknowledged that the level of maternal and fetal surveillance may be inevitably increased and the recourse to medical intervention will have a lower threshold. However, the presence of and potential for complications do not necessarily mean that women cannot achieve a normal, intervention-free labour and birth, if that is their preference. Or, alternatively, if intervention is clinically required, a normalizing of the experience through strategies often reserved for 'low-risk' women could be facilitated.

Together with increasing intervention rates, there have been national and global concerns regarding the treatment of childbearing women by their caregivers, which should always be respectful and dignified. The White Ribbon Alliance (2011) and the Care Quality Commission (2013) have acknowledged that this is not always the case. There is some evidence that dignity and respect are more evident when women give birth at home or in birth centres than when giving birth in a hospital (Birthrights Dignity in Childbirth Forum, 2013).

What is normal birth and what is challenging or complex birth?

The difficulties of defining 'normal birth' are well documented in the literature (Downe et al., 2001; MCWP, 2007; Walsh et al., 2008; Walsh and Downe, 2010) (see Box 1.1). What is considered normal childbirth in high-income, well-resourced westernized cultures is problematic. This is because in the current context of maternity care, technological interventions are commonplace and have themselves been absorbed into routine care. Taylor (2001) describes this as the 'usual' becoming the 'normal'. The boundaries between normal birth and medicalized birth have become blurred. This is supported by Downe and colleagues' (2001) study in which one-third of 956 women who gave birth in a consultant-led unit, had their births recorded as being normal or spontaneous, when in fact they had experienced induction or acceleration of labour. Downe et al. (2001) question the provenance of the terms 'normality' and 'normal birth'. This centres on whether 'normal' is the birth of the baby vaginally without the aid of instruments (despite interventions that may have occurred during labour), an entirely natural physiological process, or the common experience of women, where the notion of 'normal' really means 'usual'.

Box 1.1: Definitions of normal birth, normal delivery, spontaneous vaginal birth/delivery

Normal birth/delivery: 'one where a woman commences, continues and completes labour physiologically at term' (RCM, 2008: 1).

Normal birth/delivery: 'without induction, without the use of instruments, not by caesarean section and without general, spinal or epidural anaesthetic before or during delivery' (MCWP, 2007: 1).

Spontaneous vaginal birth/delivery: 'not assisted by forceps, vacuum, or caesarean section and not a malpresentation' (SOGC, 2008: 1163). This is what is generally reported in national statistics as the normal birth rate.

The different definitions present a challenge. Health Episode Statistics (2012) report that in 2011–2012, approximately 61.2% of women in England had a 'spontaneous vaginal birth'. However, when using the Maternity Care Working Party (MCWP) definition of 'normal birth', the rate is 41.8% (Dodwell and Gibson, 2014). In response to the issue of 'normal birth rates' being reported inconsistently, Miranda Dodwell and Rod Gibson (2014) (who developed the BirthChoiceUK website) now report normal birth rates in line with the MCWPs's definition. When comparing different maternity units in England in 2011, the highest normal birth rate was reported as 54% and the lowest at 28.8% (Dodwell and Gibson, 2014). Interventionist childbirth is clearly now becoming the norm.

Challenging or complex childbirth may be even more difficult to define and indeed can be subjective depending on one's philosophical view of childbirth and familiarity with the evidence base. For example, conducting searches on breech,

I found many references to this being 'abnormal' but others would describe it as being 'unusual'.

Indeed, in the latest edition of *Myles Textbook for Midwives* (Marshall and Raynor, 2014), breech appears in the physiology and care during first and second stages of labour chapters rather than in the traditional 'malpresentations' chapter (Downe and Marshall, 2014; Jackson et al., 2014). This is because the editors and authors have a view that breech in itself is not inherently 'abnormal'. Definitions of complex or complicated pregnancy, labour or birth in the literature are difficult to find. This is presumably because the terms are quite wide and may cover many conditions affecting childbearing women. However, Wildschut (2011: 11) defines a high-risk pregnancy as follows: 'the probability of an adverse outcome for the mother or child is increased over and above that of the baseline risk of that outcome among the general population by the presence of one or more ascertainable risk factors or indicators'. Wildshut (2011) goes on to assert that this definition does not account for the significance or degree of the risk, or the relevance of the health outcome to the general childbearing population.

Case 1.1: Karen

The idea for this book was conceived in 1995, although I did not realize it at the time. I was pregnant with my daughter and although everything during the pregnancy was straightforward, the labour and birth became more complex. At 39 + 4 weeks' gestation, my waters broke one morning but no contractions started. After waiting for over 24 hours, having a Clary Sage massage and then Prostin per vaginum, still nothing happened. I eventually went to the labour suite where intravenous Syntocinon was commenced at 16.30 hours.

My midwife (and best friend) Barbara examined me at 20.30 and found my cervix to be 3 cm dilated. With my forewaters intact, she conducted an artificial rupture of membranes (ARM) and a 'sweep' and I immediately felt the contractions more intensely. I coped for another two hours and then I completely lost it. The contractions were very strong and extremely painful. When you hear women say, 'I can't do it', 'I want to go home', 'can I have a caesarean?' – I really relate to that now. The phrase that I thought of was 'please shoot me through the head'. I truly would have done anything to relieve that pain. At 22.30, cervix still 3 cm, I had an epidural that was difficult to insert but once in, gave me fantastic relief. At 02.30 the next morning, my cervix was found to be fully dilated; I was so relieved, I cried, whatever happened now it was almost certainly going to be a vaginal birth. I pushed well to start with, but as the epidural wore off a little at the fundus, I could feel this little foot in my rib, which stopped me from pushing effectively. Eventually, the Senior Registrar on duty came in to give me a little helping hand. She applied the ventouse cup, pulled Megan down a little and around the curve of Carus, and then did something I had never heard of before – she took the cup off her head, to enable me to push her out and Barbara 'delivered' Megan at 07.55 (see Figure 1.1). Everyone was crying, my mum, my partner, Gabriel, Barbara, Megan, even the Senior Registrar – it was a magical moment.

The reason I have included my own story is, looking back, every step of the way efforts were made by everyone involved in my care to make my childbearing experience as 'normal' and as humanized as possible. Every decision was made by me and respected and supported by the doctors and midwives. Enabling me to push Megan out to have at least a part 'normal birth' (as I viewed it at the time) was really important to me physiologically and psychologically. It was also hugely significant for Barbara, to 'deliver' Megan after she had so kindly and patiently cared for me for all those many hours. I know it wasn't easy for her seeing me in pain. Though my childbirth experience was not what I would have planned, I consider it to be a very wonderful and very positive event in my life.

With permission of Megan and Barbara.

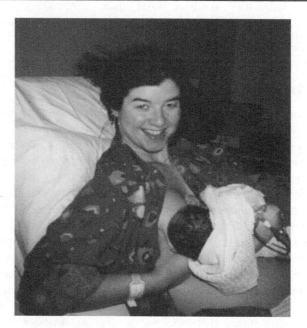

Figure 1.1

Reflection points

- Have you witnessed obstetricians (or midwives) take off a ventouse cup, or forceps, before crowning has occurred?
- Could this approach be discussed and explored within your unit?
- How could this be aired with your obstetric colleagues?
- Would you, one of your colleagues or one of your students be interested in this aspect of birth as a research project?

Although I am aware that some practitioners do remove a ventouse cup or forceps blades just prior to 'crowning' in some circumstances, it is not something I personally have witnessed. I asked the Normal Birth Research Group (normal-birth-research@jiscmail.ac.uk) for any information, literature or evidence surrounding this practice. Some midwives, including those in Scandinavian countries, stated that this was common practice in their units. However, the only literature that I could find that included a description of this was Byrom and colleagues' (2010) wonderful story of a mother who had experienced a traumatic birth first time around and was desperate not to have a repeat caesarean section. After hours of pushing, it became clear she needed some help. With her in a standing position, the obstetrician used the ventouse to pull the infant down by about a centimetre. She then pushed out the head and the body spontaneously and felt completely elated. She said that the obstetrician had ensured she left the hospital not as a patient but as a mum. It seems an intuitive and simplistic strategy to humanize the birth process, thus it is surprising to find very little literature relating to this practice.

Models of childbirth

Accompanying the shift to hospital birth, there has been a philosophical shift from a social model of childbirth to a biomedical model and this has had a major impact on the experience of childbearing for women (van Teijlingen, 2005; Walsh, 2012). The most often quoted difference between these philosophical viewpoints is that the medical model only sees pregnancy and childbirth as normal in retrospect, whereas the social model of childbirth sees pregnancy and childbirth as a normal physiological event. There are other fundamental differences between these two contrasting models (see Table 1.1, also refer to Table 3.1), but Walsh (2012) makes the point that in modern maternity practice, few obstetricians would be seen to be completely adopting a biomedical ethos and not all midwives embrace a social model of care. Although there is an overlap and blurring of the divisions, the model remains a valuable heuristic tool for illustrating the core differences in approaches to childbirth. In the context of challenging or complex childbirth, it seems entirely appropriate and even desirable for these models, which essentially are in opposition, to blend to arrive at the correct approach and care for childbearing women. Thus taking into consideration the obstetric or medical requirements, together with individualized holistic care, while respecting women's choices and decision-making.

The hegemony of a biomedical model can be illustrated by the continuous rise in intervention during childbirth, including rates of induction of labour, epidurals, instrumental deliveries and caesarean section rates in the UK (Health Episode Statistics, 2012). In contrast, Davis-Floyd and Davis (1996) describe medical interventions in maternity care as the 'technocratization' of birth. They propose that the medical profession views women's bodies as defective and that their pregnant bodies will become more efficient when attached to more perfect diagnostic machinery. They suggest that there appears to be a cultural

Table 1.1 Medical model and social/midwifery model of childbirth.

Medical model	Social/midwifery model
Doctor-centred	Woman-centred
Objective	Subjective
Male	Female
Body–mind dualism	Holistic
Pregnancy and childbirth: only normal in retrospect	Pregnancy and childbirth: normal physiological process
Statistical/biological approach	Individual psycho-social approach
Biomedical focus	Psycho-social focus
Medical knowledge is exclusionary	Knowledge is not exclusionary
Intervention	Observation
Public	Private
Outcome: aims for live, healthy mother and baby	Outcome: aims for live, healthy mother and baby and satisfaction of individual needs of mother/couple
Control and manage	Respect and empower
Homogenization	Celebrate difference
Technology as partner	Technology as servant

Sources: Davis-Floyd and Sargent (1997), Oakley (1999), van Teijlingen (2005), Walsh (2012).

supervaluation of machines over bodies and technology over nature (Davis-Floyd and Davis, 1996).

The deconstruction of birth and the subsequent debates surrounding hospital versus home (Gyte et al., 2010; Wax et al., 2010), abdominal versus vaginal birth (NICE, 2011), medicalization versus holism (Walsh, 2012), are all relatively recent developments, with some claiming that technological childbirth makes birth safer (RCOG, 2008). Yet, there is good evidence from well-conducted research studies and Cochrane systematic reviews, that technocratic birth is only appropriate for women at risk of complications where the intervention(s) would benefit mother, fetus or both. It has been suggested that technocratic childbirth may be associated with women feeling deprived of power and control over their own bodies (Davis-Floyd and Davis, 1996; Green et al., 2003; Stewart, 2004; Stewart et al., 2004; Walsh and Downe, 2010; Birthplace in England Collaborative Group, 2011; Hodnett et al., 2012). However, it must also be acknowledged that some 'low-risk' childbearing women make informed choices to embrace technology during labour and birth (McIntosh, 2012), and that some do choose to bypass vaginal birth altogether and make an informed decision to have a caesarean section delivery; however, the number of women requesting caesarean section without medical indication is very small (McCourt et al., 2004). In contrast, some childbearing women in the 'high-risk' category make informed decisions to have little or no medical intervention. The motivation for this appears to be past negative experiences of maternity services.

A recent history of maternity care in the UK

The introduction of the National Health Service (NHS) in 1948 was a significant landmark in British history and is associated with improvements in maternal and neonatal health (Louden, 2000). However, in terms of reducing maternal mortality, there was dramatic change prior to the introduction of the NHS, which Louden (2000) attributes mainly to highly trained, experienced midwives caring for pregnant women with uncomplicated pregnancies largely at home (see Figure 1.1). Hospital care by obstetricians was reserved for women with complicated pregnancies.

From 1950, maternal and neonatal mortality continued to decrease. In 1954, the neonatal mortality rate was 18 per 1000 live births; in 1997, it was 5.3 per 1000 live births (CEMACH, 2006) and by 2009 it had fallen to 3.2 per 1000 live births (CMACE, 2011). Maternal mortality also decreased dramatically (see Figure 1.2), with obstetricians stating that the move to hospitalized birth was the reason (Louden, 2000). This view did not take into account that women's general health was improving, that they were having fewer babies because of contraception, that housing conditions were also improving, and overcrowding was becoming less of a problem (Campbell and Macfarlane, 1994; Tew, 1998). In addition, from the 1930s, antibiotics were being used to treat puerperal sepsis, and infection control was becoming more prominent (Humphries and Bystrianyk, 2013). In other words, improvements in public health could, in part, explain the decreases. Louden (2000) also cites the use of ergometrine, blood transfusions, antibiotics, better training, better anaesthesia, improved organization of maternity services and less interference in normal labours as reasons contributing to the overall decline in maternal mortality rates.

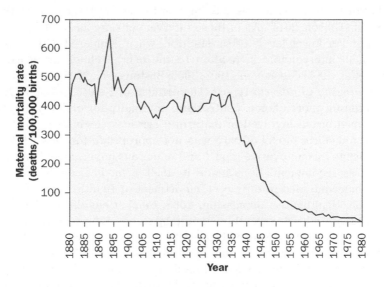

Figure 1.2 Maternal mortality in England and Wales.

Source: Adapted from Louden (2000).

As early as the late 1950s, a discourse was developing which claimed that in addition to physical health, emotional and psychological health was just as important for the overall wellbeing of childbearing women (Morris, 1960). This suggestion continues to appear in health policy, most notably in *Changing Childbirth* (Department of Health, 1993) and every subsequent maternity policy, including the most recent national maternity review: Better Births (Cumberlege 2016). During the 1960s, midwifery had been viewed as an 'art'-based profession, in contrast to obstetrics, which positioned itself very much as a 'science'. This coincided with technological advances such as ultrasound scanning. During this and the subsequent decade, the concept of 'scientific birth' emerged, wherein science was seen as capable of controlling nature, including childbirth (McIntosh, 2012).

In 1970, the Peel Report recommended that the resources of modern medicine should be available to all mothers and babies, and that sufficient facilities should be provided to allow for 100% hospital delivery (Ministry of Health, 1970). Although this recommendation was for 100% 'availability' of resources, hospital birth rates soared without any evidence to support this fundamental change in health policy. In addition, no one asked mothers if they wanted to give birth in hospitals (Beech, 2006). The alternating impetus from pressure groups (and indeed from midwives) initially campaigning for hospital births and access to pain relief, then back again to home and natural birth is a paradox that cannot be adequately explored here. This issue is comprehensively discussed by McIntosh (2012), who suggests that it was middle-class, well-educated women who initially lobbied for change, including access to hospital birth, not necessarily taking account of the wishes of the invisible group of working-class, non-articulate childbearing women.

As the rates of women giving birth in acute institutions increased, so did medicalization of the childbearing process. Interventions such as induction, epidurals and assisted births have all risen substantially over the last 50–60 years (see Table 1.2) (Dodwell and Gibson, 2014). All of these interventions are associated with higher morbidity and/or lower levels of satisfaction, when compared with labours and births without intervention, in relation to the overall childbearing experience (Glazener et al., 1995; Green et al., 1998, 2003; Baston et al., 2008).

The *Changing Childbirth* report (Department of Health, 1993), with its recommendation for more choice, control and continuity for childbearing women, was welcomed by all involved in maternity services (McIntosh, 2012). It also stated that a medical model of care was not appropriate for most childbearing women. Despite this innovative report and numerous government health reports endorsing the recommendations made in 1993, a medical model approach to childbirth has continued to develop (Department of Health, 2004, 2007a 2007b, 2010a, 2010b; Healthcare Commission, 2008, Cumberlege 2016). The legacy of *Changing Childbirth* was recently revisited by many of those originally involved with its publication (McIntosh and Hunter, 2013). It is acknowledged that it was a groundbreaking report which should have made a positive impact on maternity service development. In many ways it failed to do so, but the underpinning philosophy of *Changing Childbirth* fundamentally to humanize maternity care for all childbearing women is just as relevant today as when it was published more than 20 years ago.

Table 1.2 Mode and place of birth, instrumental and epidural rates.

	1955	1990	2009	2011
Home birth rate (England and Wales)	33.4	1.0	2.9	2.4
NHS hospital birth rate (England and Wales) (%)	60.2	97.9	96.5	97.6
Induction rate (England) (%)	13.0	18.4	20.2	21.3
Caesarean rate (England) (%)	2.2	11.3	24.6	24.8
Instrumental rate (England) (%)	4.4	9.4	12.1	12.5
Epidural rate (England) (%)	—	17.0	33.0	36.0

Source: Dodwell and Gibson (2014).

The maternity services have yet to demonstrate lower intervention rates and increased normal births. Paradoxically, intervention rates have increased, even in normal straightforward childbirth (Walsh, 2012).

Normalizing childbirth and organizational models of care, birth environment and place of birth

Birth centres and midwife-led care units are primarily for 'low-risk' childbearing women, thereby excluding women with more challenging or complex pregnancies. Case-holding midwifery models, where the same midwife or small group of midwives cares for a pregnant woman throughout the childbearing process, generally regardless of 'risk', are thought to provide a more woman-centred approach to maternity care (McCourt, 2010). There are a number of case-holding practices in the UK that report increased vaginal/normal birth rates, lower intervention rates, lower caesarean section rates and improved satisfaction rates for women, compared with 'traditional' or 'usual' care (Andrews et al., 2006; McCourt, 2010). As an illustration, Table 1.3 lists some differences between caseload outcomes and national average outcomes for aspects of maternity care, for Southampton City Primary Care Trust.

Early studies found that in contrast to traditional models of care, childbearing women of different risk status were statistically more likely to know their carer (Page et al., 1999; North Staffordshire Changing Childbirth Research Team, 2000; Benjamin et al., 2001), and have fewer interventions such as induction of labour (Benjamin et al., 2001) and augmentation of labour (North Staffordshire Changing Childbirth Research Team, 2000) when part of a case-holding scheme. Epidural use was also reduced (Page et al., 1999; North Staffordshire Changing Childbirth Research Team, 2000). Expectant mothers were also statistically more likely to have a home birth, give birth in a midwife-led unit, have a normal birth, as well as more likely to opt for an early discharge home (Benjamin et al., 2001).

Tracey et al. (2013) conducted a controlled trial in two teaching hospitals in Australia in which 871 pregnant 'all-risk' women were randomized to caseload midwife-led care and 877 to standard care. Although the maternal and neonatal

Table 1.3 Maternity outcomes for caseload care in Southampton City Primary Care Trust.

Outcome	Caseload care (%)	National rates (%)
Vaginal birth rate	68	62
Breastfeeding rate	83	70
LSCS rate	17	23
Preterm births	3.9	7
Smoking rate	13	19.5

Source: Nelson (2010).

outcomes were similar in the two groups, the caseload model was significantly less expensive than the standard care. The authors concluded that caseload midwifery is safe and cost-effective for childbearing women irrespective of risk factors.

A Cochrane review by Sandall et al. (2015) examined midwife-led models of care compared with medical-led or shared care. The review included fifteen trials including 17,674 women of both low risk and increased risk of complications. The midwife-led care model showed a reduction in epidural use, episiotomies and instrumental deliveries. Women in this model were also more likely to have a spontaneous vaginal birth and know the midwife who cared for them during labour. There were also less pre-term births and fewer overall fetal/neonatal deaths. No adverse effects were found for the midwife care model. There were no significant differences in caesarean section rates or intact perineums.

Given the known benefits and improved outcomes from caseholding models of maternity care, it could be argued that when women are offered this option, the potential for normalized labour and birth are maximized. The stark reality is that most women in the UK give birth in acute healthcare settings, and receive care from a midwife who is unknown to them (Birthplace in England Collaborative Group, 2011).

Continuous care in labour (Hodnett et al., 2013), having a known midwife during care in labour (Page et al., 1999), non-supine positions during labour (Lawrence et al., 2009) and a shared philosophy of normal birth (Kennedy et al., 2004) have all been shown to increase normal/spontaneous vaginal birth rates and reduce unnecessary interventions. All these aspects of care are more likely to occur in midwife-led units or at home.

Case 1.2: Casey

Casey was a 17-year-old primigravida, who came to the labour suite accompanied by her 17-year-old boyfriend. She appeared to be in established labour and therefore after the midwife conducted the usual professional duties, Casey was encouraged to mobilize around the labour suite. They were a very 'mature' couple and her boyfriend seemed to instinctively know how to support her.

After a few hours, Casey's contractions were becoming increasingly intense and regular and she requested to go into the pool. Unfortunately, the pool was out of use, so I suggested the next best thing. I filled the bath and, upon entering, she immediately relaxed and it became clear that she did not want to get out of the water. I discussed her wishes for the birth including the third stage of labour. Although she did not want any injections (mainly because of a fear of needles), her haemoglobin was 9.9 g/dL (as recorded then), just below accepted levels in the guidelines for a physiological third stage. I explained the potential risks and benefits but she insisted that she did not want any interference, which included injections.

Casey gave birth to a very healthy boy, who went straight to the breast, the placenta delivered spontaneously very quickly afterwards, and blood loss was minimal, approximately 50 mL. Mother and father were ecstatic at how amazing they found the birth experience. The midwife who took over from me was far from impressed that she had had a physiological third stage considering her haemoglobin status. I explained that everything had been thoroughly discussed with the woman (and her partner) and that I'd supported her in her decision, documenting everything in the notes.

Practice points

- Would you support a woman in making a decision like this, even if this might go against your own feelings, or against the local 'guidelines'?
- Would you back up a midwife colleague who supports a woman with a decision that might not adhere to local guidelines?

Rising intervention rates

It is clear that intervention rates in childbirth are increasing and that normal birth rates are as a consequence falling. In 1985, the spontaneous vaginal birth rate in England was 75.4% and the caesarean section rate 10.4%; in 2011–12, the spontaneous vaginal birth rate had fallen to 61.2% and the caesarean section rate had risen to 25% (see Table 1.2) (Health Episode Statistics, 2012; Dodwell and Gibson, 2014). The increase of operative deliveries in the last 30 years has not been accompanied by any measurable improvement in outcomes for babies, such as hypoxic ischaemic encephalopathy (Institute for Innovation and Improvement, 2006; NICE, 2011).

In 1990, the epidural rate was 17% and the induction rate 18.4%. By 2011, the epidural rate had risen to 36% and the induction rate to 21.3% (see Table 1.2). The use of appropriate technology in childbirth when there are complications is sometimes necessary to reduce morbidity and mortality. However, the use of technology should be clearly medically justified. This is because birth without medical intervention is associated with much less pain during the postnatal period (Johanson et al., 1993; Glazener et al., 1995), a faster physical recovery from the birth (Johanson et al., 1993; Glazener et al., 1995), an increase in self-esteem (Llewelyn and Osborne, 1990), enhanced bonding with the baby (Odent, 1999; Ferguson et al., 2002), a reduced likelihood of postnatal depression (Fisher et al., 1997; Green et al., 2003), a calmer, more settled baby (Kitzinger, 1989) and a better breastfeeding experience (Odent, 1999) than a medicalized birth. Glazener et al. (1995) concluded that the optimal mode of delivery in terms of health outcomes is usually a normal vaginal birth, with both caesarean section and instrumental delivery more likely to be associated with residual maternal morbidity at one year. Moreover, Green et al. (1998, 2003) and Baston et al. (2008) found that higher levels of obstetric interventions were an important factor in predicting negative experiences of childbirth.

Caesarean section versus normal birth

It is clear that for some childbearing women who experience a complicated pregnancy/labour, a caesarean section will be the safest mode of delivery. However, it is also clear that in the absence of clinical need, and in the knowledge of some of the disadvantages of caesarean section, some women still choose this mode of birth. There is the obvious convenience of knowing when and where a baby is going to be born and the relative short time frame for delivery by caesarean section. These seem to be the main advantages of caesarean section delivery reported by women (NICE, 2011). Lavender et al. (2009) attempted a review but found no trial data to reach any conclusions regarding the superiority of one mode of birth over the other. However, the same authors also highlighted the urgent need for a review of observational and qualitative studies to compare normal vaginal birth with caesarean section in terms of health outcomes for mother and baby.

There is ongoing debate about the relative advantages and disadvantages of normal birth and caesarean section, which cannot be given justice here. The literature reviewed would appear to suggest that, compared with vaginal birth, caesarean section delivery has higher associated maternal morbidity rates (Institute for Innovation and Improvement, 2006; NICE, 2011) and higher maternal mortality rates (Hall and Bewley, 1999; Wen et al., 2004), although NICE (2011) does state that the evidence surrounding maternal mortality is complex and equivocal. Some studies cite higher neonatal morbidity rates (Fogelson et al., 2005) and higher neonatal mortality rates (MacDorman et al., 2008). In addition, caesarean sections are twice as expensive as normal or vaginal births (NICE, 2011). The inference of these findings is, therefore, that caesarean section should be reserved for maternal and/ or fetal conditions that warrant this mode of birth. Finally, there is a concern that some childbearing women are not making real choices about their labours and births, and are not being involved in decisions regarding the use of technology in their childbirth experience, which may make them more likely to elect a caesarean mode of delivery (Baston et al., 2008).

Conclusion

There is an abundance of evidence to support a more normalized approach to child-birth, even when there are challenges or complexities involved (Institute for Inno-vation and Improvement, 2006, 2007; Healthcare Commission, 2008; Mead, 2008; Davis-Floyd, 2011). Different approaches, models, and ways of organizing mater-nity care (Kennedy et al., 2004; Hodnett et al., 2013; Sandall et al., 2015) can support a more normalized approach in all risk categories of childbirth. When women are provided with good quality information, continuity of carer and one-to-one support in labour, they tend to follow a more normality-focused labour and birth experi-ence, rather than relying on unnecessary intervention or technology (McCourt et al., 2006; Lawrence et al., 2008; Hodnett et al., 2012).

Further reading

BirthChoiceUK website [http://www.birthchoiceuk.com/Professionals/index.html]. This web-site, created by Miranda Dodwell and Rod Gibson Associates Ltd., provides the most up-to-date maternity information and statistics using the MCWP definition of 'normal birth'.

McCourt, C., Stevens, T., Sandall, J. and Brodie, P. (2006) Working with women: developing continuity of care in practice, in R. McCandlish and L. Page (eds) *The New Midwifery: Science and sensitivity in practice* (2nd edn.). London: Elsevier. Provides a discussion on the positive aspects and development of continuity of care in the maternity services.

Sandall, J., Soltani, H., Gates, S., Shennan, A. and Devane, D. (2015) Midwife-led continuity models versus other models of care for childbearing women, *Cochrane Database of System-atic Reviews*, 9: CD004667. Demonstrates the effectiveness of midwife led models of care when compared to obstetrician led models of care for childbearing women.

References

Andrews, S., Brown, L., Bowman, L., Price, L. and Taylor, R. (2006) Caseload midwifery: a review, *Midwifery Matters*, 108 (Spring): 15–20.

Baston, H., Rijnders, M., Green, J. and Buitendijk, S. (2008) Looking back on birth three years later: factors associated with a negative appraisal in England and in the Netherlands, *Journal of Reproductive and Infant Psychology*, 26 (4): 323–39.

Beech, B. (2006) At last – an NMC home birth circular, *AIMS Journal*, 18 (1) [http://aims.org.uk/Journal/Vol18No1/NMCHomebirthCircular.htm].

Benjamin, Y., Walsh, D. and Taub, N. (2001) A comparison of partnership caseload midwifery care with conventional team midwifery care: labour and birth outcomes, *Midwifery*, 17: 234–40.

Birthplace in England Collaborative Group (2011) Perinatal and maternal outcomes by planned place of birth for healthy women with low risk pregnancies: the Birthplace in England national prospective cohort study, *British Medical Journal*, 343: d7400.

Birthrights Dignity in Childbirth Forum (2013) *Dignity in Childbirth. The Dignity Survey 2013: Women's and midwives' experiences of UK maternity care* [http://www.birthrights.org.uk/wordpress/wp-content/uploads/2013/10/Birthrights-Dignity-Survey.pdf].

Byrom, S., Fardella, J., Sandford, J., Martindale, L., Barden, L. and Theophilou, G. (2010) Col-laborating to push boundaries to promote positive birth: an inspirational reflection, *MIDIRS Midwifery Digest*, 20 (2): 199–204.

Campbell, R. and Macfarlane, A.J. (1994) *Where to be Born? The debate and the evidence* (2nd edn). Oxford: National Perinatal Epidemiology Unit.

Care Quality Commission (2013) *National Findings from the 2013 Survey of Women's Experiences of Maternity Care* [https://www.cqc.org.uk/sites/default/files/documents/maternity_report_for_publication.pdf].

Centre for Maternal and Child Enquiries (CMACE) (2011) *Perinatal Mortality 2009: United Kingdom*. London: CMACE [http://www.publichealth.hscni.net/sites/default/files/Perinatal%20Mortality%202009.pdf].

Confidential Enquiry into Maternal and Child Health (CEMACH) (2006) *Perinatal Mortality Surveillance Report, 2004: England, Wales and Northern Ireland*. London: CEMACH [http://www.sepho.org.uk/Download/Public/10056/1/PMR2004_March2006.pdf].

Cumberlege, J. (2016) *Better Births: Improving outcomes of maternity service in England*. The National Maternity Review england.maternityreview@nhs.net www.england.nhs.uk/ourwork/futurenhs/mat-review.

Davis-Floyd, R. (2011) The technocratic, humanistic and holistic paradigms of childbirth, *International Journal of Gynaecology and Obstetrics*, 75 (suppl. 1): S5–S23.

Davis-Floyd, R. and Davis, E. (1996) Intuition as authoritative knowledge in midwifery and home birth, in R. Davis-Floyd and C. Sargent (eds) The Social Production of Authoritative Knowledge in Childbirth, *Medical Anthropology Quarterly*, 10 (2): 237–69.

Davis-Floyd, R. and Sargent, C. (eds) (1997) *Childbirth and Authoritative Knowledge: Cross-cultural perspectives*. Berkeley, CA: University of California Press.

Department of Health (1993) *Changing Childbirth: Report of the Expert Maternity Group* (Cumberlege Report). London: HMSO.

Department of Health (2004) *National Services Framework for Children, Young People and Maternity Services*. London: Department of Health.

Department of Health (2007a) *Maternity Matters: Access, choice and continuity of care in a safe service*. London: Department of Health.

Department of Health (2007b) *Making it Better: For mother and baby*. London: Department of Health.

Department of Health (2010a) *Equity and Excellence: The government strategy to liberate the NHS*. Norwich: TSO.

Department of Health (2010b) *Midwifery 2020: Delivering expectations*. London: Department of Health.

Dodwell, M. and Gibson, R. (2014) *Normal Birth Rates in Scotland and England* [www.birthchoiceuk.com; accessed 31 August 2014].

Downe, S. and Marshall, J. (2014) Physiology and care during the transition and second stage phases of labour, in J.E. Marshall and M.D. Raynor (eds) *Myles Textbook for Midwives* (16th edn). Edinburgh: Churchill Livingstone.

Downe, S., McCormick, C. and Beech, B. (2001) Labour interventions associated with normal birth, *British Journal of Midwifery*, 9 (10): 602–6.

Downe, S. and McCourt, C. (2008) From being to becoming: reconstructing childbirth knowledges, in S. Downe (ed.) *Normal Childbirth Evidence and Debate* (2nd edn). London: Churchill Livingstone.

Ferguson, J., Young, L. and Insel, T. (2002) The neuroendocrine basis of social recognition. *Frontiers in Endocrinology*, 23 (2): 200–4.

Fisher, J., Astbury, J. and Smith, A. (1997) Adverse psychological impact of operative obstetric interventions: a prospective longitudinal study, *Australia and New Zealand Journal of Psychiatry*, 31 (5): 728–38.

Fogelson, N., Menard, M., Hulsey, T. and Ebeling, M. (2005) Neonatal impact of elective repeat cesarean delivery at term: a comment on patient choice cesarean delivery, *American Journal of Obstetrics and Gynecology*, 192 (5): 1433–6.

Glazener, C., Abdalla, M., Stroud, P., Naji, S., Templeton, A. and Russell, I. (1995) Postnatal maternal morbidity: extent, causes, prevention and treatment, *British Journal of Obstetrics and Gynaecology*, 102: 282–7.

Green, J., Baston, H., Easton, S. and McCormick, F. (2003) *Greater Expectations: Inter-relationships between women's expectations and experiences of decision making, continuity, choice and control in labour, and psychological outcomes*. Summary report. Leeds: Mother & Infant Research Unit, University of Leeds.

Green, J., Coupland, V. and Kitzinger, J. (1998) *Great Expectations: A prospective study of women's expectations and experiences of childbirth*. Hale: Books for Midwives Press.

Gyte, G., Dodwell, M., Newburn, M., Sandall, J., MacFarlane, A. and Bewley, S. (2010) Findings of meta-analysis cannot be relied on, *British Journal of Medicine*, 341: c4033.

Hall, M. and Bewley, S. (1999) Maternal mortality and mode of delivery, *Lancet*, 335: 776.

Healthcare Commission (2008) *Towards Better Births*. London: Commission for Healthcare Audit and Inspection.

Health Episode Statistics (2012) *Method of Delivery 1980–2009/2010: NHS Hospitals England*. Health and Social Care Information Centre [http://www.statistics.gov.uk/hub/health-social-care/specialist-health-services/maternity-and-pregnancies-services; accessed 15 August 2013].

Hodnett, E., Downe, S. and Walsh, D. (2012) Alternative versus conventional institutional settings for birth, *Cochrane Database of Systematic Reviews*, 8: CD000012.

Hodnett, E., Gates, S., Hofmeyr, G. and Sakala, C. (2013) Continuous support for women during childbirth, *Cochrane Database of Systematic Reviews*, 7: CD003766.

Humphries, S. and Bystrianyk, R. (2013) *Dissolving Illusions. Disease, vaccines and the forgotten history*. Create Space Independent Publishing [online].

Institute for Innovation and Improvement (2006) *Focus On: Caesarean section*. Coventry: NHS Institute for Innovation and Improvement.

Institute for Innovation and Improvement (2007) *Pathways to Success: A self improvement toolkit – focus on normal birth and reducing caesarean rates*. Coventry: Coventry: NHS Institute for Innovation and Improvement.

Jackson, K., Marshall, J. and Brydon, S. (2014) Care during the first stage of labour, in J.E. Marshall and M.D. Raynor (eds) *Myles Textbook for Midwives* (16th edn). Edinburgh: Churchill Livingstone.

Johanson, R., Wilkinson, P., Bastible, A. Ryan, S., Murphy, H. and O'Brien, S. (1993) Health after childbirth: a comparison of normal and assisted delivery, *Midwifery*, 9 (3): 161–8.

Kennedy, H., Shannon, M., Chuahorm, U. and Kravetz, K. (2004) The landscape of caring for women: a narrative study of midwifery practice, *Journal of Midwifery and Women's Health*, 49 (1): 14-23.

Kitzinger, S. (1989) *The Crying Baby*. London: Penguin.

Kitzinger, S. (2000) *Rediscovering Birth*. London: Simon & Schuster.

Kitzinger, S. (2005) *The Politics of Birth*. Edinburgh: Elsevier Butterworth Heinemann.

Lavender, T., Hofmeyr, G., Neilson, J., Kingdon, C. and Gyte, G. (2009) Caesarean section for non-medical reasons at term, *Cochrane Database of Systematic Reviews*, 3: CD004660.

Lawrence, A., Lewis, L., Hofmeyr, G., Dowswell, T. and Styles, C. (2009) Maternal positions and mobility during first stage labour, *Cochrane Database of Systematic Reviews*, 2: CD003934.

Lawrence Beech, B. and Phipps, B. (2008) Normal birth: women's stories, in S. Downe (ed.). *Normal Childbirth: Evidence and debate* (2nd edn.). Edinburgh: Churchill Livingstone.

Llewelyn, S. and Osborne, K. (1990) *Women's Lives*. London: Routledge.

Louden, I. (2000) Maternal mortality in the past and its relevance to developing countries today, *American Journal of Clinical Nutrition*, 72 (1): 241–6.

MacDorman, M., Declercq, E., Menacker, F. and Malloy, M. (2008) Neonatal mortality for primary Cesarean and vaginal births to low risk women: application of an intention to treat model. *Birth*, 35 (1): 3–8.

Marshall, J.E. and Raynor, M.D. (eds) (2014) *Myles Textbook for Midwives* (16th edn). Edinburgh: Churchill Livingstone.

Maternity Care Working Party (MCWP) (2007) *Making Normal Birth a Reality*. London: Royal College of Midwives, Royal College of Obstetricians and Gynaecologists, National Childbirth Trust.

McCourt, C. (2010) How midwives should organise to provide intrapartum care, in D. Walsh and S. Downe (eds) *Essential Midwifery Practice: Intrapartum care*. Chichester: Wiley-Blackwell.

McCourt, C., Bick, D. and Weaver, J. (2004) Caesarean section: perceived demand, *British Journal of Midwifery*, 12 (7): 412–14.

McCourt, C., Stevens, T., Sandall, J. and Brodie, P. (2006) Working with women: developing continuity of care in practice, in R. McCandlish and L. Page (eds). *The New Midwifery: Science and sensitivity in practice* (2nd edn.). London: Elsevier.

McIntosh, T. (2012) *A Social History of Maternity and Childbirth: Key themes in maternity care*. London: Routledge.

McIntosh, T. and Hunter, B. (2013) 'Unfinished business'? Reflections on changing childbirth twenty years on, *Midwifery*, 30 (3): 279–81.

Mead, M. (2008) Midwives – practices in three European countries, in S. Downe (ed.) *Normal Childbirth: Evidence and debate* (2nd edn.). London: Churchill Livingstone.

Ministry of Health (1970) *Domiciliary Midwifery and Maternity Bed Needs: Report of the Standing Maternity and Midwifery Advisory Committee* (Sub-committee Chairman J. Peel). London: HMSO.

Morris, N. (1960) Human relations in obstetric practice, *Lancet*, 1 (7130): 913–15.

National Institute for Health and Clinical Excellence (NICE) (2011) *Guidelines for Caesarean Section*. London: NICE.

Nelson, J. (2010) Caseload midwifery – does it improve outcomes?, *MIDIRS Midwifery Digest*, 20 (3): 309–11.

North Staffordshire Changing Childbirth Research Team (2000) A randomised study of midwifery caseload care and traditional 'shared care', *Midwifery*, 16: 295–302.

Oakley, A. (1999) Who cares for women? Science versus love in midwifery today, in E. van Teijlingen, G. Lowis, P. McCaffery and M. Porter (eds) *Midwifery and the Medicalization of Childbirth: Comparative perspectives*. New York: Nova Science.

Odent, M. (1999) *The Scientification of Love*. London: Free Association Books.

Page, L., McCourt, C., Beake, S., Vail, A. and Hewison, J. (1999) Clinical interventions and outcomes of one-to-one midwifery practice, *Journal of Public Health Medicine*, 21 (3): 243–8.

Royal College of Midwives (RCM) (2008) *Campaign for Normal Birth: Definitions and the RCM position paper* [http://www.rcmnormalbirth.org.uk/default.asp?sID=1103625596157; accessed 29 July 2013].

Royal College of Obstetricians and Gynaecologists (RCOG) (2008) *Standards for Maternity Care*. London: RCOG.

Sandall, J., Soltani, H., Gates, S., Shennan, A. and Devane, D. (2015) Midwife-led continuity models versus other models of care for childbearing women, *Cochrane Database of Systematic Reviews*, 9: CD004667.

Society of Obstetricians and Gynaecologists of Canada (SOGC) (2008) Joint Policy Statement on Normal Childbirth, *Journal of Obstetrics and Gynaecology Canada*, 30 (12): 1163–5.
Stewart, M. (2004) *Pregnancy, Birth and Maternity Care: Feminist perspectives*. London: Elsevier Science.
Stewart, M., McCandlish, R., Henderson, J. and Brocklehurst, P. (2004) *Review of Evidence of Clinical Psycho-social and Economic Outcomes for Women with Straightforward Pregnancies who Plan to Give Birth in a Midwife-led Birth Centre, and Outcomes for their Babies: Report of a structured review of birth centre outcomes*, December 2004 – Revised 2005. Oxford: National Perinatal Epidemiology Unit [https://www.npeu.ox.ac.uk/downloads/files/reports/Birth-Centre-Review.pdf].
Taylor, D. (2001) What is usual? Normality in maternity care, *British Journal of Midwifery*, 9 (6): 390–3.
Tew, M. (1998) *Safer Childbirth? A critical history of maternity care*. London: Chapman & Hall.
Tracey, S., Hartz, D., Tracy, M., Allen, J., Forti, A., Hall, B. et al. (2013) Caseload midwifery care versus standard maternity care for women of any risk: M@NGO, a randomised controlled trial, *Lancet*, 382 (9906): 1723–32.
van Teijlingen, E. (2005) A critical analysis of the medical model as used in the study of pregnancy and childbirth, *Sociological Research Online*, 10 (2).
Walsh, D. (2012) *Normal Labour and Birth: A guide for midwives* (2nd edn). London: Routledge.
Walsh, D. and Downe, S. (eds) (2010) *Essential Midwifery Practice: Intrapartum Care*. Chichester: Wiley-Blackwell.
Walsh, D., El-Nemer, A. and Downe, S. (2008) Rethinking risk and safety in maternity care, in S. Downe (ed.) *Normal Childbirth: Evidence and debate* (2nd edn). London: Churchill Livingstone.
Wax, J., Lucas, F., Lamont, M., Pinette, M., Cartin, A. and Blackstone, J. (2010) Maternal and newborn outcomes in planned home birth vs. planned hospital birth: a metasynthesis, *American Journal of Obstetrics and Gynaecology*, 203 (3): 243e1–243e8.
Wen, S., Rusen, I., Walker, M., Liston, R., Kramer, S., Baskett, T. et al. (2004) Comparison of maternal mortality and morbidity between trial of labor and elective cesarean section among women with previous cesarean delivery, *American Journal of Obstetrics and Gynecology*, 191 (4): 1263–9.
White Ribbon Alliance (2011) *Respectful Maternity Care: The Universal Rights of Childbearing Women Charter* [http://whiteribbonalliance.org/wp-content/uploads/2013/10/Final_RMC_Charter.pdf].
Wildschut, H. (2011) Constitutional and environmental factors leading to a high risk pregnancy, in D. James, P. Steer, C. Weiner, B. Gonik, C. Crowther and S. Robson (eds) *High Risk Pregnancy: Management options*. St Louis, MO: Saunders.

2

Positive approaches to health for childbearing women

Karen Jackson

Mother Theresa stated that she would not participate in a march against war but would participate if the march were for peace.

Wilmington College (undated)

Introduction

Midwives are often quoted as being the guardians of normal births. While this is essentially true, it is also well documented that complexity in childbirth is increasing (Raynor, 2012; Knight et al., 2014). This is due to a number of factors, including increasing maternal age, increased levels of obesity and increasing numbers of women with diabetes (Knight et al., 2014), all of which will inevitably have an effect on maternity services provision. In addition, women with medical conditions such as cardiomyopathy, renal disease and some haemoglobinopathies are choosing to become mothers, when even 20 years ago, pregnancy may have been actively discouraged or even considered life-threatening. Women's mental health and social welfare are also seemingly more complex, which is apparent in contemporary maternity services. And because of reproductive technologies, multiple births are more common. Breech presentations rarely result in a vaginal birth. Both multiple pregnancy and breech presentation are generally considered to be 'high risk'.

A major challenge in caring for women with complex childbearing issues is in helping them to achieve a positive, as well as safe, childbirth experience. These women can become caught between the dichotomy of obstetric and midwifery philosophies. Obstetrics is a medicalized discipline, established on the study of disease and disorders and a concomitant quest to reduce risk. Midwifery is based on a presumption of normality, but also recognizing that deviations from the norm can and do occur. Women who find themselves labelled as obstetric cases have more medical appointments and are often less likely to have access to midwives. These two perspectives have the potential to lead to discord, and that is more likely when pregnancy and childbirth are challenging or complex. There is also the potential that the label of complexity can lead to the assumption that the birth will be completely medicalized, and that the mother's choices will be limited. A complex pregnancy should not mean that opportunities to access less medicalized care are reduced. While health professionals are well aware of the risks associated with all of the conditions mentioned above, women can still achieve an optimal birth experience, which can be 'normalized' and 'humanized' in accordance with her wishes and in line with what is feasible and appropriate. Concepts of health such as salutogenesis, resilience and optimality resonate well with challenging and complex childbirth in the quest to focus on enabling rather than disabling factors. The quote at the beginning of this chapter illustrates perfectly the emphasis on positive rather than negative discourses, and all these constructive approaches will be discussed in this chapter. Other emerging ideas and approaches will also feature.

The dominant health discourse of 'risk' in maternity care

Much of healthcare is heavily medicalized: the study of disease and disorder. Midwifery is one discipline that seeks to distance itself from this, as pregnancy and birth inherently recognized as a normal, physiological process. The introduction of risk factors can tip the balance into pathogenesis, potentially making the fit and healthy pregnant woman a 'patient' in need of 'treatment'. By subtly changing the attitude of the care provider, ensuring that information is delivered appropriately, the risk can often be managed without needing to be medicalized, but the fear of adverse outcomes can taint the experience (Schmid and Downe, 2010). It is of course difficult to separate risk and outcome, and is especially emotionally charged in midwifery. The whole notion of 'risk' can itself have an adverse effect on women and on maternity services more generally (see Chapter 3). Indeed, some suggest using 'chance' rather than 'risk', as the latter is laden with negative connotations.

It is rare to find a practitioner – midwife or doctor – who sits at either end of the sliding scale between completely medicalized and wholly midwifery-led. Practice and experiences influence perceptions and opinions of how pregnancy and birth can progress. Workplace culture, and in particular exposure to a medicalized environment, have been found to adversely affect risk perception in midwives, leading to an overreliance on intervention, and a lack of trust in the natural processes of childbirth (Mead and Kornbrot, 2004). If there is a perceived high risk, information presented to women about their choices may echo that, perhaps leading these women to believe that they need to follow a more interventionist path (Mead and Kornbrot, 2004). It is now well recognized that there is a need for more humanization in higher risk pregnancy, to counterbalance and normalize as much as possible (Wagner, 2001; Behruzi et al., 2010). The burden of responsibility that the healthcare practitioner (HCP) carries, as a licensed practitioner, can affect the way information is presented.

The very label of 'complex' or 'high risk' can make women feel inadequate, and while it should be seen as a marker for specialist care, it can also be used as a tool for controlling women (Tracy, 2006). It can also be very subjective. Some HCPs may view a relatively benign deviation from the norm as 'risk'; for example, ketosis in labour can be rectified easily by encouraging hydration and appropriate nutrition.

For some practitioners, however, this would immediately trigger the siting of an intravenous infusion, with the subsequent effect of limiting or reducing mobility.

Medical appointments are often more frequent and can become focused on the medical 'problem' without regard for what is going 'right' in the pregnancy. There is a fixation with 'risk' factors rather than 'wellness' factors. Women who are having complex pregnancies may spend more time in the care of obstetricians than midwives. Sometimes it may seem impossible to find the time to talk about the things that are normal in midwifery-led care. Women may potentially miss out on vital information about feeding, preparing for birth, mental health and postnatal care (see Rachel's story in Chapter 12).

Generally, it has been found that women labelled as high risk have a more difficult experience in childbearing, including experiencing more negative emotions (Heaman and Gupton, 2009). This is likely to be in part because of their experience of increased medical surveillance during maternity healthcare, rather than or in addition to the complex nature of their pregnancy.

It is clear that stress and anxiety can have a negative impact on pregnancy and childbirth. The physiological effects of stress regulation are numerous, and outcomes can be adversely affected. Physiologically, it has been found that anxiety during labour is associated with high levels of the stress hormone epinephrine in the blood, which can lead to abnormal fetal heart rate patterns, inefficient uterine contractility, a longer active labour phase and low neonatal Apgar scores (Lederman et al., 1978; Lederman et al., 1981).

Regulating stress and anxiety should be a priority in all labours but especially so in challenging and complex cases. To overcome the constant message of 'risk', which can translate to childbearing women as 'danger', requires skill and sensitivity by the midwife. It is also prudent to be aware that the stress that the caregiver experiences can affect outcomes as well – either directly, through an over-cautious approach, or indirectly, by adversely affecting the stress levels of the woman and her family (Schmid and Downe, 2010).

What is 'salutogenesis'?

When deconstructed from Latin, salutogenesis means 'origins of health'. The western medical model is rooted in pathogenesis – the study of disease rather than wellbeing. Pathogenesis works retrospectively from disease to determine how individuals can avoid, manage and/or eliminate that disease. Salutogenesis works prospectively by considering how to create, enhance and improve physical, mental and social wellbeing (Becker et al., 2010: 1). Antonovsky (1979) postulated that in traditional healthcare models there is no possibility of individuals with chronic conditions achieving wellbeing – health cannot co-exist with disease. Except that, this is not the case, and through his body of work Aaron Antonovsky (1979, 1987) hypothesized that the origins of health could be accessed through a 'sense of coherence'. This central concept of the salutogenic model states that a sense of wellbeing is intrinsically linked with a strong sense of self and desire to achieve wellness. A sense of coherence has three component parts: comprehensibility, manageability and meaningfulness (see Box 2.1).

Box 2.1: A sense of coherence

Comprehensibility: Understanding the world (or a particular problem) and being able to make sense of it.

Manageability: Having sufficient internal and/or external resources to cope.

Meaningfulness: Believing that life, or a particular event, has purpose.

Source: After Antonovsky (1979, 1987).

Much of midwives' work is about encouraging a sense of self-belief in mothers-to-be and their pregnant bodies. To maintain that encouragement when there are challenges can be difficult, but this is where the salutogenic model proves useful. As Antonovsky (1979) said, we share a commitment to understand and enhance the adaptive capacity of human beings. For midwives, it is exhilarating to enable and empower a woman to achieve more than she thought she was capable of.

Antonovsky postulated his theory in relation to survivors of concentration camps following the Second World War; he pondered why they had survived such a traumatic experience when others perished or were left scarred psychologically. The answer appeared, in part, to be related to attitude. Those who could embrace positivity, even in these darkest of times, appeared more resilient.

In the field of psychology and mental health, a focus on salutogenesis has been explored as an alternative approach to traditional therapy concentrating on previous adverse life events. Langeland et al. (2007) discussed three healing factors that have been suggested to be important in the recovery process for mental health clients (Strauss, 1996; Anthony et al., 2002). These factors are that participants: (1) perceive themselves as something other than just a diagnosis and a disease; (2) explore themselves with respect to their whole person; and (3) take control of their own lives (Langeland et al., 2007: 276). It is clear to see that these factors are just as applicable to other areas of healthcare, including maternity.

Case 2.1: Nessa

Nessa was a self-confident and bright woman who had lost her first child when her uterus ruptured at 22 weeks. Following consultation with healthcare professionals, and after carefully considering the risks, she was happy to be pregnant again, but understandably nervous. The midwifery and obstetric teams worked closely together with Nessa, and agreed a schedule of increased appointments to monitor for any concerns. The midwifery appointments had a relaxed and informal feel, and concentrated on Nessa's psychological wellbeing as much as her physical state. She had remarkable resilience, and had a sunny disposition despite the risk that surrounded her pregnancy. Control, or the lack of it, dominated her thoughts, so the midwifery care concentrated on the aspects that Nessa could influence. She ate well, and took early maternity leave when it seemed that work was adversely affecting her. She also started expressing milk at 28 weeks for an anticipated delivery at 32 weeks, although it was not until 34 weeks that her son was delivered via caesarean section. Through her own research Nessa sought to normalize the birth, and asked for delayed cord clamping if possible, and early skin to skin for her or her partner. Her son had a brief visit to the neonatal intensive care unit for assessment, before being reunited with his mother and they both recovered well. Postnatally, Nessa reported a sense of achievement, accomplishment, and pride in the birth and how she was able to bond with her son. It is likely that Nessa had a strong sense of coherence.

Resilience

It is interesting to note that the term 'resilience' is often cited in literature exploring salutogenesis. Resilience is the ability to successfully withstand a threatening and challenging situation. It also refers to recovery from extreme distress and trauma (Agaibi and Wilson, 2005). Many definitions of resilience refer to successful or positive adaptation to adversity (Luthar et al., 2000). From a conceptual perspective, resilience is associated with curiosity and intellectual skills and the ability to deal with problems (Block and Kremen, 1996; Agaibi and Wilson, 2005).

In some illuminating research, Hunter and Warren (2013) explored resilience in midwifery. Despite rising birth rates, increasing complexity in childbearing, staff shortages, low morale and high stress levels, some midwives had long and fulfilling careers in midwifery and indeed remained positive and motivated throughout. Seery et al. (2010) add that this adaptation is without residual significant psychological or physiological disruption. Hunter and Warren (2013: 7) conclude that: 'resilience is the ability of an individual to respond positively and consistently to adversity, using effective coping strategies'. This concept appears to be closely allied to salutogenesis. If the principles of resilience can be taught, learned, promoted or facilitated, the implications for midwives and for childbearing women are obvious.

There is evidence that resilience, through psycho-education, can indeed be taught or promoted but to date most studies have not been randomized (Saisto et al., 2006). In one study (Salmela-Aro et al., 2011), nulliparous women with a self-rated severe fear of childbirth were randomized into either an intervention group ($n = 131$) or a control group ($n = 224$). The intervention was a series of six psycho-education sessions during pregnancy and one following the birth. The sessions included the promotion of resilience and a sense of mastery to enable the women to cope should any 'setbacks' occur during labour or birth. Such strategies were presumed to enhance positive motherhood following the birth (Salmela-Aro et al., 2011). The intervention increased women's preparedness for childbirth, which also predicted an increase in positive motherhood. The authors conclude that the results are promising and that resilience can be strengthened (Salmela-Aro et al., 2011).

Case 2.2: Gemma

Gemma, aged 27, was a survivor of childhood sexual abuse. She experienced horrendous abuse around the age of 11. She disclosed her abuse when she became an adult after previously having had intensive counselling. She had become a very successful businesswoman, was very sociable, with a very likeable personality and a well-developed sense of humour. Gemma and her husband Ben had a very close and loving relationship. She did state that she was a self-confessed control freak.

Gemma was pregnant with her first child and had reached full term without any issues. However, she had met with one of the midwifery team beforehand and stated that in labour she wanted everything to be explained to her and that she wanted to be involved in any decisions to be made. She underwent a series of edu- cational sessions (psycho-education), in preparation for the labour and birth. Gemma also had a detailed birth plan, which expressed a desire for few if any vaginal exam- inations but that if these became necessary, the caregiver had to provide a clear rationale for them and that they should be conducted gently and with sensitivity.

Gemma's labour progressed slowly and at one point an audible deceleration was heard via the Pinard stethoscope. The attending midwife felt that it was necessary to conduct a vaginal examination to assess progress. At Gemma's request, she wanted to sit in a more semi-recumbent position rather than lying recumbent on the bed. Gemma also asked to feel and touch a pair of latex gloves, prior to the examination. Following a discussion between them, the mid- wife touched Gemma's leg and then thigh with her gloved hand, before gently examining her, explaining everything that she was doing, reassuring her that she would stop the examination at any time.

The midwife then explained her findings to Gemma in detail. Fortunately, labour was well advanced and Gemma soon gave birth to a healthy baby girl. Gemma and Ben were ecstatic and Gemma stated that she really appreciated the kind and compassionate care she had received.

Despite Gemma's childhood ordeals, she had developed an optimistic per- sonality, and was clearly a high-achieving, happy, functioning adult. She demon- strated incredible resilience and felt that the educational sessions she had attended had helped her to 'cope' and not 'lose it' when it seemed at one point that the labour was not going to plan.

Optimality

Kennedy defines optimality thus: 'Optimality, specifically defined for perinatal health care, is the maximal perinatal outcome with minimal intervention placed against the dynamic context of the woman's social, medical, and obstetric history' (2006: 766). In a concept analysis of optimality in maternity care, Kennedy (2006) found that optimality is an appropriate conceptual label for a care approach in the maternity services that promotes and supports the physiological processes of childbirth without unjustified technologic or obstetric intervention. This concept is not just confined to normal, 'low-risk' women but can be applied to all risk categories – meaning that any woman can achieve an optimal birth in her particular circumstances.

Romano (2007) examined four studies that supported the promotion of normality over technology, thereby increasing women's optimality in childbirth. In the first, Cragin and Kennedy (2006) assigned 196 women with moderate risk factors, defined as three or more medical or psycho-social risk factors, to midwife-led care and another 179 women to an obstetric-led group. They found that compared with obstetric-led care, midwifery-led care increased optimality significantly. For example, the caesarean section rate was 13% in the midwife-led group and 34% in the physician-led care. In a second study, Gaudernack et al. (2006) conducted a randomized controlled trial (RCT) and reported that acupuncture ($n = 48$) administered following pre-labour rupture of membranes reduced length of labour and oxytocin use compared with the group ($n = 52$) that did not receive acupuncture. Third, Fitzgerald et al. (2007) compared 407 primigravid women who sustained anal sphincter tears with 390 women who did not sustain such tears. They reported a strong relationship between obstetric practices such as episiotomy, epidural use and instrumental vaginal delivery and increased anal sphincter tears. They suggested that these interventions are modifiable, whereby possible vacuum extraction rather than forceps should be used and episiotomy avoided. Finally, Beebe and Humphreys (2006), in an in-depth ethnographic analysis of 23 childbearing women's experiences, concluded that a reassessment is required of how childbirth educators teach women to self-diagnose labour. In addition, introducing home visits, providing out-of-hospital early-labour assessment and ensuring women feel supported, may help women who choose hospital birth to optimize the timing of hospitalization to achieve a normal birth. The review of these four studies demonstrates that promoting normality, empowering women through education and reducing interventions in childbirth, all increase optimality for women.

Practice point

Many maternity units hold inter-professional meetings such as cardiotocography (CTG) meetings, or perinatal morbidity/mortality forums that essentially review incidents and practices that may have led to sub-optimal outcomes. Could you foster an approach in your maternity unit that focuses on the positive aspects of childbearing women's health such as normal birth meetings that review incidents and practices that resulted in positive outcomes?

Other positive approaches to childbirth

Darra (2009) adopts a postmodernist view of the terminology 'normal birth'. A normal or natural birth, she believes, may not be appropriate to promote, given the very unique experience of childbirth for each and every woman. Indeed, she sees Downe's (2004) theory of 'unique normality' and Armstrong's (1983) 'normal variability' as more useful for contemporary childbearing women. Humanizing the birth process may also be preferable to the promotion of 'normality', as the very definitions of 'normal' and 'normality' are hotly contested (see Chapter 1). Darra (2009) embraces the pragmatic concept of 'the good enough birth' (akin to the psychological theories put forward in the 1950s and 1960s of the 'good enough mother'). Although she articulates and argues her standpoint extremely well, being entirely practical and rational, it does raise the issue of women (and by association, midwives) being contented with feeling that they have had a birth that is merely considered 'good enough'. While a 'good enough birth' might be grounded in the reality of modern-day expectations and experiences of maternity care, surely the aspiration is to have an empowering, amazing, life-affirming birth.

At a time when the traditional teaching of relaxation at antenatal classes is waning, a number of positive approaches to childbirth have emerged. Mindfulness, hypnobirthing, neurolinguistic programming, yoga and the Alexander technique are all strategies that help women to develop a positive, confident, powerful outlook on childbirth. This in turn has helped to prepare women for the challenges of labour and birth by empowering them to deal with any issues in a constructive way. At present, little in the way of a sound evidence base exists to support the success or otherwise of these approaches. In a Cochrane review, Madden et al. (2012) stated that hypnotherapy showed promise in relation to reducing pain in labour and thus reducing the need for other interventions, but recommended that more research be conducted. Hopefully an evidence base – whether qualitative or quantitative – will develop rapidly to endorse these more empowering, woman-centred approaches to childbirth.

Respectful inter-professional relationships and their role in humanizing childbirth

There is clearly a role for midwives and obstetricians in the care of women with challenging or complex needs. Many reports have highlighted effective inter-professional relationships to be key in improving safe care for mothers and babies (HCC, 2006; NICE, 2007; NPSA, 2007; CMACE, 2011; Thomas and Dixon, 2012). Where there is poor communication, discord and disrespect, this can lead to dysfunctional team working. This not only potentially affects the care of childbearing women and their babies, but possibly increases morbidity and mortality rates too (Downe, 2010; CMACE, 2011; Thomas and Dixon, 2012; Kirkup, 2015). As midwives and obstetricians will be all too aware, the devastating effects of dysfunctional team working was starkly exemplified in the recent Kirkup Report (2015).

However, safety is not the only consideration. There is increasing emphasis on the importance of equal and respectful collaborations between the disciplines involved in maternity care (Downe, 2010). Where teams have mutual respect, trust and have friendly working relationships, high-quality care is enhanced, as reported by women themselves (Ontario Women's Health Council, 2006, cited in

Downe, 2010). Such an environment engenders job satisfaction, which ultimately transfers to women. The positive approaches to health for childbearing women are pertinent here.

Conclusion

This chapter has examined some of the more positive, constructive approaches to health and wellbeing in childbirth rather than the predominant risk and fear discourses that prevail in maternity care. Salutogenesis, resilience and optimality are all gaining in popularity with their emphasis on wellness rather than illness, positivity rather than negativity, and a sense of empowerment and achievement rather than failure and distress. Promoting normality and/or a humanized birth experience fits better with these woman-centred approaches and vice versa. Other progressive approaches such as mindfulness and hypnotherapy are emerging in maternity care but are yet to gain any substantial evidence-based validation. Finally, the best possible experience for all childbearing women can only be achieved through respectful inter-professional relationships.

Further reading

Downe, S. (2012) Skilled help from the heart: the story of a midwifery research programme, *Evidence Based Midwifery*, 10 (1): 4–9. Recounts Soo Downe's interest in salutogenesis, and how it can be applied to childbirth.

Warriner, S., Dymond, M. and Williams, J. (2013) Mindfulness in maternity, *British Journal of Midwifery*, 21 (7): 520–2. Discusses how mindfulness helps individuals to live in the present moment rather than thinking about the past or worrying about the future.

References

Agaibi, C. and Wilson, J. (2005) Trauma, PTSD and resilience: a review of the literature, *Trauma Violence Abuse*, 6 (3): 195–216.
Anthony, W., Cohen, M., Farkas, M. and Gagne, C. (2002) *Psychiatric Rehabilitation* (2nd edn). Boston, MA: Boston University, Center for Psychiatric Rehabilitation.
Antonovsky, A. (1979) *Health, Stress and Coping*. San Francisco, CA: Jossey-Bass.
Antonovsky, A. (1987) *Unraveling the Mystery of Health: How people manage stress and stay well*. San Francisco, CA: Jossey-Bass.
Armstrong, D. (1983) *Political Anatomy of the Body: Medical knowledge in the twentieth century*. Cambridge: Cambridge University Press.
Becker, C., Glascoff, M. and Felts, M. (2010) Salutogenesis 30 years later: where do we go from here?, *International Electronic Journal of Health Education*, 13: 25–32.
Beebe, K. and Humphreys, J. (2006) Expectations, perceptions, and management of labor in nulliparas prior to hospitalization, *Journal of Midwifery and Women's Health*, 51 (5): 347–53.
Behruzi, R., Hatem, M., Goulet, L., Fraser, W., Leduc, N. and Misago, C. (2010) Humanized birth in high risk pregnancy: barriers and facilitating factors, *Medicine, Health Care and Philosophy*, 13: 49–58.

Block, J. and Kremen, A. (1996) IQ and ego-resilience: conceptual and empirical connections and separateness, *Journal of Personality and Social Psychology*, 70 (2): 349–61.

Centre for Maternal and Child Enquiries (CMACE) (2011) Saving mothers' lives – Reviewing maternal deaths to make motherhood safer: 2006–2008. The Eighth Report of the confidential enquiries into maternal deaths in the United Kingdom, *BJOG: An International Journal of Obstetrics and Gynaecology*, 118 (suppl. 1): 1–203.

Cragin, L. and Kennedy, H. (2006) Linking obstetric and midwifery practice with optimal outcomes, *Journal of Obstetric, Gynaecologic and Neonatal Nursing*, 35 (6): 779–85.

Darra, S. (2009) Normal, natural, good or good enough birth: examining the concepts, *Nursing Inquiry*, 16 (4): 297–305.

Downe, S. (2004) *Normal Childbirth: Evidence and debate*. London: Churchill Livingstone.

Downe, S. (2010) Towards salutogenic birth in the 21st century, in D. Walsh and S. Downe (eds) *Essential Midwifery Practice: Intrapartum care*. Chichester: Wiley-Blackwell.

Fitzgerald, M., Weber, A., Howden, N., Cundiff, G. and Brown, M. (2007) Risk factors for anal sphincter tear during vaginal delivery, *Obstetrics and Gynecology*, 109 (1): 29–34.

Gaudernack, L., Forbord, S. and Hole, E. (2006) Acupuncture administered after spontaneous rupture of membranes at term significantly reduces the length of birth and use of oxytocin: a randomized controlled trial, *Acta Obstetricia et Gynecologica*, 85 (11): 1348–53.

Health Care Commission (HCC) (2006) *Investigation into 10 Maternal Deaths at, or following Delivery at Northwick Park Hospital, Northwest London Hospitals NHS Trust between April 2002–April 2005* [http://webarchive.nationalarchives.gov.uk/20060502043818/ http://healthcarecommission.org.uk/_db/_documents/Northwick_tagged.pdf; accessed 12 October 2014].

Heaman, M. and Gupton, A. (2009) Psychometric testing of the Perception of Pregnancy Risk Questionnaire, *Research in Nursing and Health*, 32 (5): 493–503.

Hunter, B. and Warren, L. (2013) *Investigating Resilience in Midwifery*. Final report. Cardiff: Cardiff University.

Kennedy, H. (2006) A concept analysis of optimality in perinatal health, *Journal of Obstetric, Gynaecologic and Neonatal Nursing*, 35 (6): 763–9.

Kirkup, B. (2015) *The Report of the Morecambe Bay Investigation*. London: TSO.

Knight, M., Kenyon, S., Brocklehurst, P., Neilson, J., Shakespeare, J. and Kurinczuk, J.J. (eds) (2014) *Saving Lives, Improving Mothers' Care: Lessons learned to inform future maternity care from the UK and Ireland Confidential Enquiries into Maternal Deaths and Morbidity 2009–12*. Oxford: National Perinatal Epidemiology Unit, University of Oxford [http://www.npeu.ox.ac.uk/downloads/files/mbrrace-uk/reports/Saving%20Lives%20Improving%20Mothers%20Care%20report%202014%20Full.pdf].

Langeland, E., Wahl, A., Kristoffersen, K. and Hanestad, B. (2007) Promoting coping: salutogenesis among people with mental health problems, *Issues in Mental Health Nursing*, 28: 275–95.

Lederman, E., Lederman, R., Work B. and McCann, D. (1981) Maternal psychological and physiologic correlates of fetal newborn health status, *American Journal of Obstetrics and Gynecology*, 139 (8): 956–8.

Lederman, R., Lederman, E., Work, B. and McCann, D. (1978) The relationship of maternal anxiety, plasma catecholamines, and plasma cortisol to progress in labor, *American Journal of Obstetrics and Gynecology*, 132 (5): 495–500.

Luthar, S., Cicchetti, D. and Becker, B. (2000) The construct of resilience: a critical evaluation for future work, *Child Development*, 71 (3): 543–62.

Madden, K., Middleton, P., Cyna, A., Matthewson, M. and Jones, L. (2012) Hypnosis for pain management during labour and childbirth, *Cochrane Database of Systematic Reviews*, 11: CD009356.

Mead, M. and Kornbrot, D. (2004) The influence of maternity units' intrapartum intervention rates and midwives' risk perception for women suitable for midwifery-led care, *Midwifery*, 20 (1): 61–71.

National Institute for Health and Clinical Excellence (NICE) (2007) *Acutely Ill Patients in Hospital: Recognising and responding to deterioration*. London: NICE [https://www.nice.org.uk/guidance/cg50].

National Patient Safety Agency (NPSA) (2007) *Safer Care for the Acutely Ill Patient: Learning from serious incidents*. The fifth report from the Patient Safety Observatory. London: NPSA [http://www.norf.org.uk/Resources/Documents/Resources%20documents/NPSA%20acutely%20ill%20safer%20care.pdf; accessed 12 October 2014].

Raynor, M. (2012) Recognition of the critically ill woman, in M. Raynor, J. Marshall and K. Jackson (eds) *Critical Illness, Complications and Emergencies Case Book*. Maidenhead: Open University Press.

Romano, A. (2007) Research summaries for normal birth, *Journal of Perinatal Education*, 16 (2): 47–50.

Saisto, T., Toivanen, R., Salmela-Aro, K. and Halmesmaki, E. (2006) Therapeutic group psychoeducation and relaxation in treating fear of childbirth, *Acta Obstetricia et Gynecologica*, 85 (11): 1315–19.

Salmela-Aro, K., Read, S., Rouhe, H., Halmesmaki, E., Toivanen, R., Tokola, M. et al. (2011) Promoting positive motherhood among nulliparous pregnant women with an intense fear of childbirth: RCT intervention, *Journal of Health Psychology*, 17 (4): 520–34.

Schmid, V. and Downe, S. (2010) Midwifery skills for normalising unusual labours, in D. Walsh and S. Downe (eds) *Essential Midwifery Practice: Intrapartum care*. Chichester: Wiley-Blackwell.

Seery, M., Holman, E. and Silver, R. (2010) Whatever does not kill us: cumulative lifetime adversity, vulnerability and resilience, *Journal of Personality and Social Psychology*, 99 (6): 1025–41.

Strauss, J. (1996) Subjectivity, *Journal of Nervous and Mental Diseases*, 184 (4): 205–12.

Thomas, V. and Dixon, A. (2012) *Improving Safety in Maternity Teams: A toolkit for teams*. London: King's Fund [http://www.nhsla.com/safety/Documents/Improving%20Safety%20in%20Maternity%20Services%20%E2%80%93%20A%20toolkit%20for%20teams.pdf; accessed 12 October 2014].

Tracy, S. (2006) Risk: theoretical or actual?, in L.A. Page and R. McCandlish (eds) *The New Midwifery: Science and sensitivity in practice* (2nd edn). Edinburgh: Churchill Livingstone.

Wagner, M. (2001) Fish can't see water: the need to humanize birth, *International Journal of Gynecology and Obstetrics*, 75: S25–S37.

Wilmington College (undated) Teachers Peace Resources: Peace Quotes [http://www.wilmington.edu/prcteachers/Quotes.cfm; accessed 9 November 2014].

3

Childbirth and risk

Denis Walsh

Introduction

Childbirth could be said to be in crisis across the western world. At the beginning of the twenty-first century at a time when birth has never been safer, it is increasingly rare for women to negotiate a path through labour without technology and pharmacological agents. Research has revealed the diminishing capacity for women to birth physiologically. In a major US study (Declercq et al., 2014), only 17% of women laboured without interventions such as epidurals and caesarean sections. Even in low-risk women where the focus is specifically on normal labour and birth, oxytocin to speed up labour is widely used in high-income countries and electronic fetal monitoring almost ubiquitous (Tracy et al., 2007). The vast majority of births occur in hospitals, attended by midwives and obstetricians, suggesting that women have lost faith in their own abilities to birth without this medical and professional infrastructure of support. Surrounding this context of childbirth is the pervasiveness of risk, which many believe is feeding defensive and interventionist practices in maternity care (MacKenzie Bryers and van Teijlingen, 2010; Scamell and Alaszewski, 2012). The recent launch of the *Lancet* series on Midwifery highlights the dangers of over-medicalization, not just for high-income countries but also for resource-poor nations (Renfrew et al., 2014).

This chapter explores the reasons for these trends and develops a critique of the risk discourse that, it is argued, is driving these changes in maternity services. Alternative viewpoints from sociologists, midwives and service users are discussed as a way of addressing the crisis in physiological birth. How the risk agenda can be transformed into an enabling mechanism is developed towards the end of the chapter.

The risk discourse

Risk appears all-pervasive in contemporary society, despite unprecedented levels of prosperity and technological advance in the developed world. Critics have analysed this phenomenon, particularly in relation to healthcare, and have suggested a number of characteristics to define it. These herald significant departures from earlier societies' notions of risk and health.

McLaughlin (2001) tracks a movement from risk as a neutral concept to do with probabilities of an event happening or not happening, to risk framed only as negative or undesirable outcomes. In relation to health, this movement has taken on a particular potency, fed by discourses of evidence-based medicine and health education.

Evidence-based medicine purports to reduce or eliminate risks by the appropriate use of diagnostic aids and the implementation of effective treatments. Proctor and Renfrew (2000) argue that these processes of diagnosis and treatment are predicated on quantitative research methods only, rendering more experiential, interpretive research approaches to the margins. In this way, risk is constructed exclusively in clinical terms and its management becomes a scientific matter (McLaughlin, 2001). Horlick-Jones (1998) suggest this strips risk assessment of its context-specific embeddedness and elevates the process as objective and rational. Later, it will be argued that context is essential in exploring the meaning of risk in maternity care.

Health education has shifted its emphasis away from governments and corporations providing healthy living conditions (provision of sanitation, reduction in pollutants) to the individual's responsibility for choosing healthy lifestyle options. Society is bombarded with data about the risks of certain behaviours to do with diet, exercise and sexual practices, to name but a few. The personalization of these choices imparts a moral dimension to them, so that ignoring risks is seen as irresponsible and reprehensible (Lippman, 1999).

Risk discourse and maternity care

In a number of ways, maternity care is an exemplar of the effects of the risk discourse on health. Childbirth straddles an ambiguous divide between what some perceive as an essentially physiological event and others as a pathology waiting to happen. These contrasting views have been conceptualized as emanating from differing models of care: a biomedical or technocratic model and a social model. The characteristics of these models are shown in Table 3.1 (MacKenzie Bryers and van Teijlingen, 2010).

The technocratic perspective sees birth as risky until proven otherwise. It desires preventing the worst-case scenario, regardless of the likelihood of that ever happening – an approach dubbed 'a maximum strategy' by Brady and Thompson (1981). This requires adopting a low threshold for intervening and a highly sceptical view of labour physiology. The model supervalues morbidity and mortality outcomes over all others, especially the psycho-social, and monitors outcomes by measuring what goes wrong. It also casts labouring women as patients, dependent on medical interventions to rescue them from deviations from the norm. Professional expertise and knowledge are highly sought after in this model and are considered authoritative, based on positivistic notions of objectivity, generalizability and certainty, all of which are obtained through quantitative research designs.

Table 3.1 Models of childbirth: the biomedical or technocratic model and a social model.

Technocratic/biomedical	Social
Body as machine	Whole person
Reductionism: powers, passages, passenger	Integrate: physiology, psycho-social, spiritual
Control and subjugate	Respect and empower
Expertise/objective	Relational/subjective
Environment peripheral	Environment central
Anticipate pathology	Anticipate normality
Technology as master	Technology as servant
Risk	Trust
Homogenization	Celebrate difference
Evidence	Intuition
Connection	Separation
Safety	Self-actualization

Source: MacKenzie Bryers and van Teijlingen (2010).

As the risk discourse becomes embedded in contemporary culture, so it surfaces in childbearing women, often reflected in their choices for place of birth as Chadwick and Foster (2014) recently demonstrated, with the social model aligned to home birth and the technocratic model to elective caesarean section. Chadwick and Foster's research setting was South Africa but it is worth remembering that women's request for elective caesarean section in the absence of clinical need is a marginal one within high-income countries (Kingdon et al., 2009).

Sociologists (Lauritzen and Sachs, 2001; Carolan, 2009) have typified the values of the technocratic model as belonging to the techno-rational paradigm that views science as progressive and modern. Techno-rationalism not only determines what counts as knowledge but also supports an industrial model of productivity or work. Such a view endorses efficiency and bureaucracy as fundamental to work systems. Risk assessment becomes another tool to fine-tune efficiency in labour care. Centralized provision for childbirth requires such a model and mimics assembly-line production (Perkins, 2004). This mainstream industrial model of maternity care in effect processes women through the phases of care. The organizational imperative to move women in at one end and out at the other end of hospital birth results in acute time pressures. Later in this chapter the invisibility of this organizational imperative to the risk assessment process will be explored. Labours have to be completed within a certain timeframe, and thus they are frequently accelerated if perceived to have fallen behind the clock.

Friedman's (1954) research on length of labour pathologized long labours, creating a clinical imperative for time restrictions despite question marks about the robustness of his methodology (Walsh, 2012). However, accelerating labour often leads to other interventions, such as unnecessary vaginal examinations (Scamell and Stewart, 2014). This is the territory of iatrogenesis, highlighted over 30 years ago by Illich (1977). He warned of the dangers of iatrogenesis and childbirth's recent history demonstrates a good example. At the beginning of the 1970s, electronic fetal monitoring was introduced to labour wards with the promise of reducing the incidence of perinatal mortality and morbidity linked to birth asphyxia. No such reduction occurred but the price that was paid was a dramatic increase in caesarean sections for fetal distress, with in some cases rates rising by up to 150% (Thacker, 1997). It was not until much later that randomized controlled trials demonstrated no advantage for this technology over intermittent auscultation of the fetal heart (Alfirevic et al., 2006).

Scenarios described above, repeated time and time again across maternity hospitals in the western world, encourage the development of a risk mindset in relation to labour and birth. Obstetrics is considered by risk assessors to be extremely vulnerable to litigation and is therefore a particular target of risk management strategies. This is because of the large settlements by maternity units for victims of cerebral palsy if they are found culpable (Fox et al., 2014). Risk management resonates with wider concerns in society about growing uncertainty and insecurity and, as already stated, reveals something of a paradox: we feel increasingly vulnerable to biological, environmental and technological developments, despite decreasing mortality and morbidity rates in western cultures.

Manuals on the rationale for risk management and its operational mechanisms rarely explore the assumptions underlying it or its philosophical antecedents, all of which contribute seminally to what could be called a 'discourse of risk' (Crawford, 2004). Crawford develops his argument regarding a disjunction between the goal of health and the 'disordered experience of its attempted achievement' (2004: 507) by identifying a number of characteristics in contemporary medical culture that contribute to a culture of fear. Some of these have strong resonance with current maternity care. Crawford writes of the growth in health education to assist individuals in their healthy lifestyle choices. As already mentioned, these focus on risks to personal health and amount to a 'pedagogy of danger'. Information to newly pregnant women can resemble this: guidance on food and beverages to eat and avoid, drugs to avoid, behaviours to change (smoking, stress-inducing), recommendations on safe places of birth (access to neonatal facilities, avoid home), early and regular contact with specialist maternity services (obstetricians). These reinforce the 'preciousness' of the pregnancy condition.

Crawford's second characteristic is the role of technologies in identifying risk factors and detecting early disease. This has spawned whole new categories of hidden pathology, predispositions and susceptibilities. Screening for fetal abnormality is a typical example. This has grown exponentially over the past 15 years on the back of increasing sophistication of ultrasound techniques. What began with early detection of neural tube defects has burgeoned into the identification of an apparently increasing number of genetic and/or hereditary conditions *in utero*. Unfortunately, in many cases diagnosis is provisional and throws up relative rather than absolute risks. This is the phenomenon of 'soft markers' (Getz and Kirkengen, 2003), which can generate anxiety and ambivalence in women who have to make vexed decisions about the appropriate course of action (Filley, 2000). Shickle and Chadwick (1994) dub this trend 'screeningitis' – the emotional inflammation and angst caused by the practice of inexact testing.

Lauritzen and Sachs (2001) develop this idea as the problematization of the normal where everyone starts out normal but is unable to secure their healthiness. Screening alerts them to the possibility of abnormality and the potential of a rare but theoretical risk of a future calamity. Everyone has a small chance of great misfortune and in effect become a 'not-yet-patient'. A cursory glance at maternity care notes reveals this potential. One UK maternity service lists over 60 risk factors for pregnancy in their history-taking page (Walsh, 2012). Evidence exists of the impact that a label of 'at risk' has on individual women, as shown in Williams and Mackey's (1999) study of women treated for preterm labour. The reality is that risk does not remain a statistic. It is 'experienced' by an individual and may well contribute towards the shaping of her identity.

The identification of risk factors in pregnancy is an inexact science, as Rowe (2010) demonstrated in her review of booking criteria utilized by various maternity services for home birth and birth centres. There was little agreement between them, probably contributing to the postcode lottery of home birth provision throughout England and Wales (NCT, 2009). Saxell's (2000) excellent review of risk-scoring tools for pregnancy revealed their poor predictability, adding to the argument that risk assessment for childbirth is a flawed endeavour.

In their critique of the meaning of numeracy in epidemiology's identification of risk, Adelsward and Sach (1996) illustrate how population-based risks are translated inappropriately to individual risk by clinicians. This has been identified as a major challenge by the medical profession, which has sought to educate clinicians about the appropriate communication of risk information (Gigerenzer and Edwards, 2003), and this is particularly relevant to obstetrics (Lyerly et al., 2007). An individual, identified as having risk factors, becomes a 'not yet ill' patient. Pregnancy already has its share of symptomless illness, as mild pregnancy-induced hypertension and intra-uterine growth restriction illustrate. The power of numeracy is that it is perceived as objective and 'true' and it therefore powerfully inscribes potential illness on the individual. The nuances of the risk discourse also invite dichotomous thinking, so that a risk is either present or absent, leading to the implication that a risk-free state exists (Adelsward and Sachs, 1996). This kind of woolly thinking reinforces the notion in maternity care that 'high-tech' hospitals are safer environments to give birth in because they can set in place measures to reduce the risks and rapidly treat the effects if they do occur.

Contextualizing risk

These critiques of how risk is conceptualized, particularly in maternity services, show how it is presented as a rational process, objectively undertaken for the greater good. This normative reading of risk obscures underlying values and beliefs that align it with scientific rationalism and the health specialism's professional projects. In fact, the medical profession's response to both risk management and evidence-based healthcare was initially equivocal, as they were perceived to undermine the profession's clinical autonomy (Harrison, 1998; Allen, 2000). McLaughlin (2001) has argued that the medical profession has appropriated the evidence agenda and risk management as a way of re-cementing their authority. She suggests they have developed the roles of evidence interpreter for complex clinical problems, and of determining risk factors and at-risk behaviours for different clinical conditions. Both roles are attempts to rehabilitate the profession's expert status, which had been buffeted by a number of high-profile mistakes, including the Shipman murders (Wilson, 2002).

Proctor and Renfrew (2000) and Lippman (1999) both argue that the current risk discourse orthodoxy is socially constructed and outline how health professionals retain the power to define and interpret it. Lippman's critique revolves around the use and abuse of 'choice' as a seminal characteristic of twenty-first century healthcare. How choices are presented reflects how risk is understood. She demonstrates how options that define choice are professionally dictated and that it is hard for consumers to introduce alternatives to those offered. Levy's (1999) research goes even further by illustrating that even within the acceptable options, midwives still 'gently steer' women towards the option the midwives are most comfortable with. For some women, the choices on offer are further circumscribed by their own paucity of resources, either to articulate their specific needs or to glean sufficient information from their carers to enable a genuine informed choice to be made. Kirkham (2004) continues to problematize the choice mantra as currently operationalized in maternity services. Drawing on disparate examples, her contributors deconstruct choice to demonstrate that, in the main, it is empty rhetoric and a placebo for policy-makers and strategists. At worst, it carefully circumscribes maternity care options and actually restricts choice for many women.

Crawford (2004) makes the astute observation that the ritual of risk as realized in medical culture makes us fear the unlikely but be unconcerned about the truly dangerous. Though paradoxical, this observation has resonance with how choices around place of birth and style of care are made in current maternity services. The discussion leads to the heart of contextualizing risk assessment. As Anderson (2004) insightfully argued, a number of known risks that operate on large labour wards are ignored by risk assessment procedures, which focus exclusively on the woman's own clinical features, rather than organizational deficiencies. These may include:

- lack of continuity of care and continuous support by midwives;
- inexperienced doctors at the start of their rotation;
- absence of expertise during the summer holidays, weekend night shifts, bank holidays;
- disagreements between midwife and obstetrician;
- inadequate handovers because of fatigue, intimidation;
- $12\frac{1}{2}$ hour shifts because midwives are too busy to have the breaks they are entitled to.

In completing her particular risk assessment for birthing on busy labour wards, Anderson adds to the above incidental other factors, such as unsupportive birth partners, bullying staff and a blame culture. Ball and colleagues (2003) had already highlighted the effects of a blame culture in their UK study exploring why midwives leave the profession. They found evidence of horizontal violence where many midwives felt under constant surveillance and feared reprisal if they made any errors. Stafford (2001) went further by suggesting that there is a current generation of 'what if' or 'just in case' midwives whose practice posture is defensive, linking this development to the ubiquity of risk. Robertson and Thomson (2014) have added to the chorus of voices asking for reform because of how risk is affecting midwives with their moving portrayal of the impact of critical incidents on midwives. Irony abounds here, as risk management strategy overtly emphasizes a 'no blame' culture as an objective.

Anderson's (2004) contribution underscores the centrality of context in undertaking risk analysis. If context is ignored, then its influences remain invisible, though they may represent the 'truly dangerous' as opposed to the potential and rare risks associated with the woman's medical history. Wagner (2001) articulates why risk assessors may miss contextual structural risks. He writes of the 'fish can't see water' syndrome; that is, if risk assessors are embedded within the organization where assessments are undertaken, then how the organization functions becomes normative. In effect, they are blinded to Anderson's factors.

Finally, to complete the critique of the risk discourse from the literature, Flynn (2002) argues that a new 'managerialism' is facilitating a control agenda by government in modern healthcare. The new managerialism has been borrowed from the private sector and is a kind of 'soft bureaucracy', both post-Fordist (a movement away from centralized bureaucratic, hierarchical models of organization) and neo-Taylorist (preoccupations with quantifying processes and outcomes of work). The former promotes devolution of responsibilities and accountabilities to local hospital level, while the latter requires a variety of measurements to be routinely collected and a number of clinical and organizational targets to be met. In this way, at local hospital level a self-regulated, self-disciplined ethos is created that essentially addresses a centrally driven agenda but ascribes full accountability for delivering it to the locality. For risk management this means that all risk strategy processes are developed and applied locally but the agenda is set by external agencies like those running the clinical negligence scheme for trusts (CNST). This powerful body indemnifies hospitals for insurance claims and is able therefore to dictate a variety of organizational and clinical standards for the hospital to fulfil prior to contractual agreement on insurance premiums. The CNST scheme reduces the premiums hospital pay if they comply with a range of clinical guidelines. Their appraisal of hospitals requires documented evidence of compliance with these. Scamell and Stewart (2014) demonstrate how midwives both comply and subvert this in the context of guidelines for labour progress by the timing of vaginal examinations – for example, delaying examinations until there are imminent signs of the second stage of labour, applying 'doing good by stealth' tactics to what they see as overly prescriptive injunctions (Kirkham, 1999).

Case 3.1: Jemma

Jemma went into labour at home and was transferred to a maternity unit without a midwifery-led unit, so was admitted to the labour ward. Over the next four hours her contractions spaced and slowed and the attending midwife recorded them as incoordinate, also noting that the cervix had dilated 1 cm over that period. She reported these findings to the labour ward lead midwife who invited a visiting consultant midwife to assess Jemma. After 30 minutes of meeting with Jemma, the consultant midwife reported back that the change in environment from home had generated anxiety in Jemma, resulting in a surge of adrenaline that had inhibited oxytocin, hence the contractions had 'gone off'. She recommended transferring Jemma back home with her community midwife, as Jemma now believed home would be a better setting to labour and birth in.

Reflection point

This is a good example of a holistic labour assessment that results in an alternative course of action to the usual artificial rupture of membranes and/or infusion of synthetic oxytocin.

Re-visioning risk in normal childbirth

In attempting to sketch out an alternative approach to risk management in maternity services, the following discussion emanates from beliefs and values of a social model of care. Deliberations are therefore based on a salutogenic or 'wellness' (see Chapter 2) perspective of pregnancy and childbirth (Downe and McCourt, 2008). A guiding principle becomes not the avoidance of risk but the promotion of efficacy. A good starting point is what evidence-based medicine tells us about care that supports physiological birth. It is a peculiar irony that the same examination of evidence sources that has been used to identify sundry risks to childbirth can also inform as to what facilitates normal labour and birth. Even more startling is the fact that positivist research designs deliver this verdict, despite Proctor and Renfrew's (2000) assertion of the limitation of evidence-based medicine when predicated solely on these methods.

Systematic reviews and other quantitative studies conclude that birthing units that exist alongside conventional labour wards and as geographically separate facilities (free-standing) reduce labour interventions in women deemed to be at low risk (Brocklehurst et al., 2011; Hodnett et al., 2012). Contributing to this low rate of intervention is probably the philosophy of care in this setting, which views labour and birth through a lens of normality. This focus on normality may also contribute to lower intervention rates in women deemed to be at higher risk, as shown by a Canadian study (Ontario Women's Health Council, 2001). In addition, women using these facilities are highly satisfied with their care. Researchers stress the centrality of a 'birth as normal' philosophy in achieving these outcomes (Esposito, 1999; Coyle et al., 2001). Esposito tells a remarkable story of a New York birth centre in capturing the power of philosophy to effect outcome. The birth centre explicitly adopted an 'active birth' approach to care that affirmed women's ability to birth without technology and medical interventions. Many of the women who came to the centre had had previous negative experience of medicalized birth but over the course of their pregnancy internalized a new vision. From a pessimistic disposition about the likelihood of experiencing a normal labour, they became expectant and positive and many went on to have very natural labours and births at the centre.

Alongside findings about the efficacy of birth centres, a substantial body of research has examined the style and type of care that contributes to non-interventionist, successful physiological birth. These findings emphasize the value of continuity of care (McCourt and Stevens, 2005) of having a midwife as a lead carer (Sandall et al., 2013) and of continuous support during labour (Hodnett et al., 2012).

These characteristics of care echo what Nolan (2002), a childbirth educator, believes to be fundamental to a proactive approach to risk management in maternity care. Her work also uses as a starting point promoting efficacy as opposed to identifying and avoiding risk. Her approach more aptly focuses on what women say are important themes in care provision, rather than what the professionals have researched. These have been identified many times by maternity service surveys and evaluations as the 3 C's – choice, control and continuity. British government policy explicitly endorsed them over two decades ago (Department of Health, 1993) and has continued to do so (Department of Health, 2007). Nolan urges us to build services around these themes, as they actually represent a preventative strategy. If combined with structural change to embrace birth centres and homebirth and the endorsement of a 'birth as normal' philosophy, then maternity services can create the conditions to realize efficacy.

An important adjunct to this refashioning of service priorities to address known benefits and efficacy of different models of care, is the explicit acknowledgement that the current large-scale, all-purpose, industrial model of labour care is failing women who anticipate having normal labour and birth. The corollary of all the research findings is that this model predisposes women to intervention and the widespread use of labour and birth technologies. The model itself has become a risk to normal birth. Contextualizing risk assessment inevitably leads to this conclusion, yet there is little evidence that this is acknowledged or influences risk decisions. In fact, the evidence points to the opposite. Midwifery units, whether alongside conventional labour wards or free-standing, have struggled to be established (Walsh and Downe, 2004), continuity of care pilot schemes have been discontinued (Walsh, 2001) and continuous support in labour remains an elusive objective for many units due to staff shortages (Smith et al., 2009).

Contextualizing risk assessment has other implications for maternity services, regarding their relationships with the institutional infrastructure of hospitals – that is, health and safety, and infection control. These bodies have jurisdiction over clinical environments and appear to predicate their risk assessment decisions on a worldview that endorses linearity, simplicity and certainty. This is a kind of 'one size fits all' approach. Objective principles of safe handling and infection control are simply transplanted into each new situation without engaging with the particular factors that define them. Downe and McCourt (2008) critique these foundations of positivist knowledge generation in maternity care, and their arguments could equally well apply here. There are again a number of anecdotal examples in maternity care where these external agencies have reduced options for women and negatively impacted on midwives' philosophy of care. Frustrating the provision of water birth because of health and safety concerns about the mobility of women and infection control worries regarding the cleaning of pools is one example. Restricting the availability of birth room props to facilitate active birth and requiring certain kinds of birth room décor when midwives want to create an ambience of home are further examples. But what of the risks of reinstalling a more clinical and less homely environment when birth centres have the reverse as an explicit objective?

Risk and safety in a birth centre

Ethnographies of birth centres and home birth reveal a contrasting language and meaning around the risk discourse (Walsh, 2006a; Cheyney, 2008; Overgaard et al., 2012). The inversion of the current orthodoxy around this topic could be said to be subversive, as the following examples reveal.

Booking rationale

A number of striking features have been reported in women's accounts around reasons for booking at home or in birth centres (Walsh, 2006a; Cheyney, 2008). One of the most obvious was the absence of references to the technocratic model of childbirth. Women did not raise concerns about 'risk' and 'safety' at the birth centre, at least not in the way that these terms are usually understood. They did not comment on an absence of doctors, epidural provision, electronic fetal monitoring, the facility for obstetric procedures like ventouse or caesarean deliveries, or an ambulance journey of at least 30 minutes if complications arose. Instead, women focused on the social (family and friends' recommendations, proximity for visiting), the environment (calm, homely, small-scale, ease of parking, absence of busyness) and the personal (welcome, friendliness, helpfulness). In fact, their response to the technocratic model was negative when they had previous experiences of birth at larger consultant units (Walsh, 2006b).

This serves to undermine the idea that evidence regarding the mortality and morbidity rates of different places of birth will be the dominant influence on women's decision-making.

Nesting instinct

The birth centre studies also revealed a shared preoccupation (midwives and women) with the birth environment. The midwives were continually honing the physical environment through regular makeovers to optimize it for birthing. Though this was clearly important for the women, an additional dimension to the environment emerged from the data – women's concern for the emotional ambience of the birth setting. This was illustrated by one woman's experience of visiting a birth centre (Walsh, 2006c). Having been greeted at the door by a member of staff holding a baby, she concluded that this was a baby-friendly place. It seemed to her '*the most natural thing in the world to find in an environment where babies are born*', though it is uncommon in large hospitals where carrying babies around is actively discouraged based on health and safety concerns. Women in the study were seeking a birth ambience characterized by compassion, warmth, nurture and love.

The focus on environmental and emotional ambience can be interpreted as characteristic of the nesting instinct. Human nesting instinct appears to seek out the right emotional ambience for childbearing, which is just as integral to establishing a protective, safe place for birth as are the immediate physical environs. The links with the previous discussion on choosing the appropriate place of birth are clear: the non-rational immediacy of decision-making when women visited the centre suggests an intuitive and rapid appraisal of emotional and environmental ambience. Similarly, it was the absence of the right emotional ambience in the other maternity units they visited (the more formal and depersonalized interactions with staff during their visits), together with their unsuitable physical environments, that turned women against them.

These findings don't actually challenge the alignment of risk and safety, as they seem to support an endorsement of the need for safety. It is the interpretation of what constitutes safety that is challenged here. Safety for these women had to do with their babies being protected rather than monitored, nurtured rather than managed, and loved rather than cared for. For many, the traditional hospital was a threat to these aspirations, so much so that they took the radical step of deliberately redefining the facility away from the language of hospital and medical care.

It may be that if service users, as Nolan (2002) urges, were the main arbiters of a risk strategy for maternity services, then it would look very different from what is currently on offer. Along with the birth centre women in this study, they might rehabilitate the homely, the social and the interpersonal aspects of the childbirth event, which have been largely dismantled by the technocratic and industrial approach. They might even change the process and outcome data so targeted at the moment on interventions like epidurals and morbidities such as caesarean section to wellness markers like physiological labour, normal birth and personal empowerment.

Communicating risk information

Plenty of guidance is currently available to help midwives share risk data with women to help them make an informed choice about their options. Absolute risks should generally be communicated using risk denominator out of 1000 (e.g. five in a thousand). This is because that benchmark has been tested for its meaningfulness to patients and represents odds that make a difference to patient decisions in healthcare. There is a risk of about 5 in a 1000 of a baby having a poor perinatal outcome in childbirth, wherever he or she is born. The Birthplace Study showed that if a nulliparous woman births at home, this risk rises to 9 in 1000. Some women may consider that an acceptable rise in risk and others may not, changing their preference accordingly. If you expressed this risk in a relative way (e.g. nearly a doubling in risk), it is clear it distorts the absolute risk and is an inappropriate way of communicating risk. Even better is to show a pictorial demonstration of this risk, which some are now recommending (Paling, 2003; Jordan and Murphy, 2009) (see Figure 3.1). Jordan and Murphy (2009) also counsel sharing the data in the opposite way, so a 9 in 1000 risk of a poor perinatal outcome at a homebirth also means that 991 out of 1000 babies will be fine.

Case 3.2: Sally

Sally was having her first baby and had decided that she wanted a home birth. Her community midwife discouraged her, stating that a recent study showed a doubling of risk to the baby if a woman had her first baby at home. Sally sought a second opinion from a caseload midwife from a neighbouring maternity service scheme who explained the relative risk implications of this choice. To Sally's surprise, the risk to the baby was very small. Only 5 in 1000 babies have a poorer perinatal outcome from birth and this increases to 9 in 1000 for first-time mothers birthing at home. The caseload midwife also mentioned that this also means that 991 babies out of 1000 will be absolutely fine if born at home to a first-time mother (see Figure 3.1). Sally requested a change of booking so she could access the caseload scheme and went ahead with her initial choice of a home birth.

Reflection point

It is very important to reflect on how you as a midwife use language to shape choice.

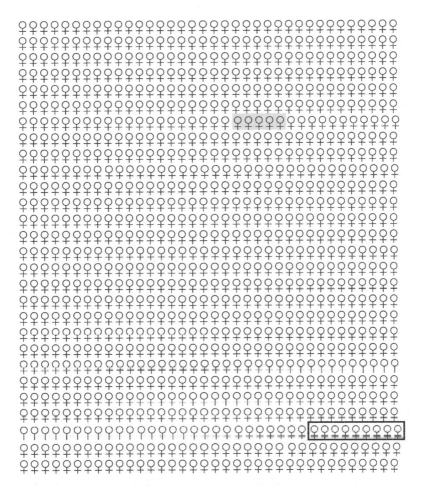

Figure 3.1 Presentation of 'risk'. A 5 in 1000 risk of uterine rupture following vaginal birth after caesarean section (VBAC) means 995 women will not have a uterine rupture following VBAC (♀). A 9 in 1000 risk of poorer perinatal outcome for primips giving birth at home means 991 babies will have a good outcome (⚲).

Source: Based on Paling's palette (2003).

Conclusion

Labour and birth care in the twenty-first century are in danger of being swamped by defensive practices emanating from an obsession with risk. The cost is in the rates of increasing childbirth interventions and in the emergence of tocophobia (fear of labour – see Chapter 5) as a psychological illness (Haines et al., 2012). There may also be long-term implications for future generations as research continues to link babies exposed to medicalized, traumatic births with destructive adult behaviours such as suicide (Jacobson and Bygddeman, 1998), eating disorders (Cnattingius et al., 1999) and drug abuse (Nyberg et al., 2000). Maternity care staff are victims as well, as adverse incidents are known to provoke stress, anxiety and even psychological harm (Robertson and Thomson, 2014).

Now is the time to take stock and to reframe avoidance of risk with likelihood of efficacy and to begin to restore confidence in physiological birth before it is too late.

Practice points

- Base your care and decisions on what is known to work best for women and normal birth – then you will maximize benefit and, by default, reduce risk.
- When sharing absolute risk information with women, give both positive and negative risks; for example, risk of caesarean scar rupture when choosing vaginal birth after caesarean section (5:1000), and the risk of not rupturing (995:1000).
- Wherever possible, share pictorial representation of risk, rather than just numerical values.
- Establishing a rapport and a relationship with women promotes a sense of trust that increases feelings of safety and security.
- Remember that language shapes experiences, so carefully select words when communicating benefits and risks.

Further reading

Dove, S. and Muir-Cochrane, E. (2014) Being safe practitioners and safe mothers: a critical ethnography of continuity of care midwifery in Australia, *Midwifery*, 30 (10): 1063–72. Provides alternative understandings that challenge traditional notions of safety.

Gigerenzer, G. and Edwards, A. (2003) Simple tools for understanding risks: from innumeracy to insight, *British Medical Journal*, 327 (7417): 741. Evidence base of alternative ways of communicating risk.

Klein, J.G. (2005) Five pitfalls in decisions about diagnosis and prescribing, *British Medical Journal*, 330 (7494): 781. Interesting reflection on non-rational clinical decision-making.

Page, M. and Mander, R. (2014) Intrapartum uncertainty: a feature of normal birth, as experienced by midwives in Scotland, *Midwifery*, 30 (1): 28–35. Provides contemporary insight into the effects of risk on practising midwives.

Walsh, D. (2006) Subverting the assembly-line: childbirth in a free-standing birth centre, *Social Science and Medicine*, 62 (6): 1330–40. Across the world, concern is being expressed about the rising rates of birth interventions. As a result, there is growing interest in alternative organizational models of maternity care. Most of the research to date on these models has examined clinical outcomes. This paper, which discusses key findings from an ethnographic study of a free-standing birth centre in the UK, explores organizational dimensions to care. It suggests that the advantages of scale have been under-recognized by policy-makers to date. The birth centre displays organizational characteristics that contrast with the dominant Fordist/Taylorist model of large maternity units. These characteristics allow for greater temporal flexibility in labour care and tend to privilege relational, 'being' care over task-orientated, 'doing' care. In addition, features of a bureaucracy are much less in evidence, enabling entrepreneurial activity to flourish. There may be lessons here for other heath services as well as maternity services in optimizing the advantages of small-scale provision.

References

Adelsward, V. and Sachs, L. (1996) The meaning of 6.8: numeracy and normality in health information talks, *Social Science and Medicine*, 43 (8): 1179–87.

Alfirevic, Z., Devane, D. and Gyte, G. (2006) Continuous cardiotocography (CTG) as a form of electronic fetal monitoring (EFM) for fetal assessment during labour, *Cochrane Database of Systematic Reviews*, 3: CD006066.

Allen, I. (2000) Challenges in the health services: the professions, *British Medical Journal*, 320 (7248): 1533–5.

Anderson, T. (2004) *The impact of the age of risk for antenatal education*, presentation to the NCT Conference, Coventry, 13 March.

Ball, L., Curtis, P. and Kirkham, M. (2003). *Why Do Midwives Leave?* London: Royal College of Midwives.

Brady, H. and Thompson, J. (1981) The maximum strategy in modern obstetrics, *Journal of Family Practice*, 12 (6): 997–9.

Brocklehurst, P., Hardy, P., Hollowell, J., Linsell, L., Macfarlane, A., McCourt, C. et al. (2011) Perinatal and maternal outcomes by planned place of birth for healthy women with low risk pregnancies: the Birthplace in England national prospective cohort study, *British Medical Journal*, 343 (7840): d7400.

Carolan, M.C. (2009) Towards understanding the concept of risk for pregnant women: some nursing and midwifery implications, *Journal of Clinical Nursing*, 18 (5): 652–8.

Chadwick, R.J. and Foster, D. (2014) Negotiating risky bodies: childbirth and constructions of risk, *Health, Risk and Society*, 16 (1): 68–83.

Cheyney, M.J. (2008) Homebirth as systems-challenging praxis: knowledge, power, and intimacy in the birthplace, *Qualitative Health Research*, 18 (2): 254–67.

Cnattingius, S., Hultman, C., Dahl, M. and Sparen, P. (1999) Very preterm birth, birth trauma, and the risk of anorexia nervosa among girls, *Archive of General Psychiatry*, 56 (7): 634–8.

Coyle, K., Hauck, Y., Percival, P. and Kristjanson, L. (2001) Ongoing relationships with a personal focus: mother's perceptions of birth centre versus hospital care, *Midwifery*, 17 (3): 182–93.

Crawford, R. (2004) Risk ritual and the management of control and anxiety in medical culture, *Health: An Interdisciplinary Journal for the Social Study of Health, Illness and Medicine*, 8 (4): 505–28.

Declercq, E.R., Sakala, C., Corry, M.P., Applebaum, S. and Herrlich, A. (2014) Major survey findings of Listening to Mothers (SM) III: new mothers speak out, *Journal of Perinatal Education*, 23 (1): 17–24.

Department of Health (1993) *Changing Childbirth: Report of the Expert Committee on Maternity Care*. London: HMSO.

Department of Health (2007) *Maternity Matters: Access, choice and continuity of care in a safe service*. London: HMSO.

Downe, S. and McCourt, C. (2008) From being to becoming: reconstructing childbirth knowledges, in S. Downe (ed.) *Normal Childbirth: Evidence and debate*. London: Churchill Livingstone.

Esposito, N. (1999) Marginalised women's comparisons of their hospital and free-standing birth centre experience: a contract of inner city birthing centres, *Health Care for Women International*, 20 (2): 111–26.

Filley, R. (2000) Obstetric sonography: the best way to terrify a pregnant woman, *Journal of Ultrasound in Medicine*, 19 (1): 1–5.

Flynn, R. (2002) Clinical governance and governmentality, *Health, Risk and Society*, 4 (2): 155–73.

Fox, R., Yelland, A. and Draycott, T. (2014) Analysis of legal claims – informing litigation systems and quality improvement, *BJOG: An International Journal of Obstetrics and Gynaecology*, 121 (1): 6–10.

Friedman, E. (1954) The graphic analysis of labour, *American Journal of Obstetrics and Gynecology*, 68 (6): 1568–75.

Getz, L. and Kirkengen, A. (2003) Ultrasound screening in pregnancy: advancing technology, soft markers for fetal chromosomal aberrations and unacknowledged ethical dilemmas, *Social Science and Medicine*, 56 (10): 2045–57.

Gigerenzer, G. and Edwards, A. (2003) Simple tools for understanding risks: from innumeracy to insight, *British Medical Journal*, 327 (7417): 741.

Haines, H.M., Rubertsson, C., Pallant, J.F. and Hildingsson, I. (2012) The influence of women's fear, attitudes and beliefs of childbirth on mode and experience of birth, *BMC Pregnancy and Childbirth*, 12 (1): 55.

Harrison, S. (1998) The politics of evidence-based medicine in the United Kingdom, *Policy and Politics*, 26 (1): 15–31.

Hodnett, E.D., Gates, S., Hofmeyr, G.J., Sakala, C. and Weston, J. (2012) Continuous support for women during childbirth, *Cochrane Database of Systematic Reviews*, 10: CD003766.

Horlick-Jones, T. (1998) Meaning and contextualisation in risk assessment, *Reliability Engineering and System Safety*, 59 (1): 79–89.

Illich, I. (1977) *Limits to Medicine. Medical nemesis: The expropriation of health*. London: Marian Boyers.

Jacobson, B. and Bygddeman, M. (1998) Obstetric care and proneness of offspring to suicide as adults: a case control study, *British Medical Journal*, 317: 1346–9.

Jordan, R.G. and Murphy, P.A. (2009) Risk assessment and risk distortion: finding the balance, *Journal of Midwifery and Women's Health*, 54 (3): 191–200.

Kingdon, C., Neilson, J., Singleton, V., Gyte, G., Hart, A., Gabbay, M. et al. (2009) Choice and birth method: mixed-method study of caesarean delivery for maternal request, *BJOG: An International Journal of Obstetrics and Gynaecology*, 116 (7): 886–95.

Kirkham, M. (1999) The culture of midwifery in the National Health Service in England, *Journal of Advanced Nursing*, 30 (3): 732–9.

Kirkham, M. (2004) *Informed Choice in Maternity Care*. London: Macmillan.

Lauritzen, S.O. and Sachs, L. (2001) Normality, risk and the future: implicit communication of threat in health surveillance, *Sociology of Health and Illness*, 23 (4): 497–516.

Levy, V. (1999) Maintaining equilibrium: a grounded theory study of the processes involved when women make informed choices during pregnancy, *Midwifery*, 15 (2): 109–19.

Lippman, A. (1999) Choice as a risk to women's health, *Health, Risk and Society*, 1 (3): 281–91.

Lyerly, A.D., Mitchell, L.M., Armstrong, E.M., Harris, L.H., Kukla, R., Kuppermann, M. et al. (2007) Risks, values, and decision making surrounding pregnancy, *Obstetrics and Gynecology*, 109 (4): 979–84.

MacKenzie Bryers, H. and van Teijlingen, E. (2010) Risk, theory, social and medical models: a critical analysis of the concept of risk in maternity care, *Midwifery*, 26 (5): 488–96.

McCourt, C. and Stevens, T. (2005) Continuity of carer: what does it mean and does it matter to midwives and birthing women?, *Canadian Journal of Midwifery Research and Practice*, 4 (3): 10–20.

McLaughlin, J. (2001) EBM and risk: rhetorical resources in the articulation of professional identity, *Journal of Management in Medicine*, 15 (5): 352–63.

National Childbirth Trust (NCT) (2009) *Homebirth Leaflet*. London: NCT.

Nolan, M. (2002) The consumer view, in J. Wilson and A. Symon (eds) *Clinical Risk Management in Midwifery: The right to a perfect baby*. Oxford: Books for Midwives Press.

Nyberg, K., Buka, S. and Lipsitt, L. (2000) Perinatal medication as a potential risk factor for adult drug abuse in a North American cohort, *Epidemiology*, 11 (6): 715–16.

Ontario Women's Health Council (2001) *Attaining and Maintaining Best Practices in the Use of Caesarean Sections* [http://www.womenshealthcouncil.com/E/index.html].

Overgaard, C., Fenger-Gròn, M. and Sandall, J. (2012) The impact of birthplace on women's birth experiences and perceptions of care, *Social Science and Medicine*, 74 (7): 973–81.

Paling, J. (2003) Strategies to help patients understand risks, *British Medical Journal*, 327 (7417): 745–8.

Perkins, B. (2004) *The Medical Delivery Business: Health reform, childbirth and the economic order*. London: Rutgers University Press.

Proctor, S. and Renfrew, M. (2000) *Linking Research and Practice in Midwifery: A guide to evidence-based practice*. London: Baillière Tindall.

Renfrew, M.J., McFadden, A., Bastos, M.H., Campbell, J., Channon, A.A., Cheung, N.F. et al. (2014) Midwifery and quality care: findings from a new evidence-informed framework for maternal and newborn care, *Lancet*, 384 (9948): 1129–45.

Robertson, J.H. and Thomson, A.M. (2014) A phenomenological study of the effects of clinical negligence litigation on midwives in England: the personal perspective, *Midwifery*, 30 (3): e121–30.

Rowe, R.E. (2010) Local guidelines for the transfer of women from midwifery unit to obstetric unit during labour in England: a systematic appraisal of their quality, *Quality and Safety in Health Care*, 19 (2). 90–4.

Sandall, J., Soltani, H., Gates, S., Shennan, A. and Devane, D. (2013) Midwife-led continuity models versus other models of care for childbearing women, *Cochrane Database of Systematic Reviews*, 8: CD004667.

Saxell, L. (2000) Risk: theoretical or actual, in L. Page (ed.) *The New Midwifery: Science and sensitivity in practice*. London: Churchill Livingstone.

Scamell, M. and Alaszewski, A. (2012) Fateful moments and the categorisation of risk: midwifery practice and the ever-narrowing window of normality during childbirth, *Health, Risk and Society*, 14 (2): 207–21.

Scamell, M. and Stewart, M. (2014) Time, risk and midwife practice: the vaginal examination, *Health, Risk and Society*, 16 (1): 84–100.

Shickle, D. and Chadwick, R. (1994) The ethics of screening: is 'screeningitis' an incurable disease?, *Journal of Medical Ethics*, 20 (1): 12–18.

Smith, A., Dixon, A. and Page, L. (2009) Health-care professionals' views about safety in maternity services: a qualitative study, *Midwifery*, 25 (1): 21–31.

Stafford, S. (2001) Is lack of autonomy a reason for leaving midwifery?, *The Practising Midwife*, 4 (7): 46–7.

Thacker, S. (1997) Lessons in technology diffusion: the electronic fetal monitoring experience, *Birth*, 24 (1): 58–60.

Tracy, S.K., Sullivan, E., Wang, Y.A., Black, D. and Tracy, M. (2007) Birth outcomes associated with interventions in labour amongst low risk women: a population-based study, *Women and Birth*, 20 (2): 41–48.

Wagner, M. (2001) Fish can't see water: the need to humanize birth, *International Journal of Gynaecology and Obstetrics*, 75 (suppl. 1): S25–S37.

Walsh, D. (2001) Birthwrite: continuity and caseload midwifery, *British Journal of Midwifery*, 9 (11): 671.

Walsh, D.J. (2006a) *Improving Maternity Services: Small is beautiful – lessons from a free-standing birth centre.* Oxford: Radcliffe Publishing.

Walsh, D. (2006b) Subverting the assembly-line: childbirth in a free-standing birth centre, *Social Science and Medicine*, 62 (6): 1330–40.

Walsh, D.J. (2006c) 'Nesting' and 'Matrescence' as distinctive features of a free-standing birth centre in the UK, *Midwifery*, 22 (3): 228–39.

Walsh, D. and Downe, S. (2004) Outcomes of free-standing, midwifery-led birth centres, *Birth*, 31 (3): 222–9.

Williams, S. and Mackey, M. (1999) Women's experience of pre-term labour: a feminist critique, *Health Care for Women International*, 20: 29–48.

Wilson, J. (2002) Clinical risk modification: a collaborative approach to midwifery care, in J. Wilson and A. Symon (eds) *Clinical Risk Management in Midwifery: The right to a perfect baby.* Oxford: Books for Midwives Press.

4

The supervisory perspective

Mary Ellen Vance

Introduction

The supervision of midwives has been enshrined in primary legislation in the United Kingdom for over 100 years. It commenced in England and Wales with the Midwives Act 1902, in Scotland with the Midwives (Scotland) Act 1915 and in Northern Ireland with the Midwives (Ireland) Act 1918. All three Acts aimed to protect the public by laying down statutory powers that included the development of systems for licensing midwives and prohibiting unqualified practice, thereby protecting women from unsafe midwifery practice.

Box 4.1: History of the development of supervision in midwifery

Although pre-dating the Universal Declaration of Human Rights, the statutory framework of supervision promotes the right to health as outlined in Article 25 (United Nations, 1948):

'(2) Everyone has the right to a standard of living adequate for the health and well-being of himself and of his family, including . . . medical [midwifery] care . . . (3) Motherhood and childhood are entitled to special care and assistance . . .'

And Article 12 of the International Covenant on Economic, Social and Cultural Rights (United Nations General Assembly 1966) states:

'1. The States Parties to the present Covenant recognize the right of everyone to the enjoyment of the highest attainable standard of physical and mental health. 2. The steps to be taken by the States Parties to the present Covenant to achieve the full realization of this right shall include those necessary for:

(a) The provision for the reduction of the stillbirth rate and of infant mortality and for the healthy development of the child; . . .
(d) The creation of conditions which would assure to all medical [midwifery] service and medical [midwifery] attention in the event of sickness'.

According to Horton (2008), the right to the highest attainable standard of health equates to the availability, accessibility, acceptability and quality of healthcare services.

This chapter will examine the role of the supervisor of midwives in supporting women with challenging or complex pregnancies when they request no or little intervention in their labours and births. First, the context of the statutory supervision of midwives in the twenty-first century will be explained, including the recent decision by the government to remove statutory supervision from the Nursing and Midwifery Council's regulatory legislation. This is followed by an exploration of the role of supervisors in promoting normality in labour and birth, the woman's right to choose, midwives' duty of care and the importance of effective communication.

Throughout, cases based on real experiences of women will be presented to demonstrate the importance of the role of the supervisor of midwives in supporting women with challenging or complex pregnancies when they request little or no intervention in their labours and births.

The context of the statutory supervision of midwives in the twenty-first century

The Nursing and Midwifery Order 2001 created the legal framework for the Nursing and Midwifery Council (NMC), which came into being in 2002. The formation of the NMC created a single, integrated, regulatory council for the whole of the UK, which has responsibility for monitoring the statutory supervision of midwives.

Although the principal aim of the statutory supervision of midwives is the protection of the public, the philosophy is centred on promoting best practice and excellence in care, preventing poor practice and intervening in unacceptable practice. This framework includes midwives who work outside of NHS organizations, such as self-employed midwives and agency midwives.

Local Supervising Authorities (LSA) are organizations within geographical areas, responsible for ensuring that the statutory supervision of midwives is undertaken according to the standards set by the NMC under Article 43 of the Nursing and Midwifery Order 2001, details of which are set out in the NMC's rules and standards for midwives (NMC, 2012b). LSA arrangements differ across the UK. In England the LSA sits within NHS England, in Scotland the LSAs are the Health Boards, in Wales the Healthcare Inspectorate is the LSA, while in Northern Ireland the Public Health Agency is the LSA.

Each LSA has an appointed LSA Midwifery Officer (LSAMO) to carry out the LSA function. The LSAMOs are practising midwives with experience in statutory supervision and provide an essential point of contact for supervisors of midwives to consult for advice on aspects of supervision. Members of the public who seek help or support concerning the provision of midwifery care can also contact the LSAMO directly. The LSA and LSAMO do not represent the interests of either provider or commissioning organizations (Bacon, 2011). This factor is a major strength in the supervisory framework and in this respect it is unique (Read and Wallace, 2014).

Supervisors of midwives are experienced midwives who have undergone additional education and training in the knowledge and skills needed to supervise midwives. They can only be appointed by an LSA, not by an employer, and act as an impartial monitor of the environment of care and the safety of midwives' practice. They are responsible to the LSA for all their supervisory activities. Supervisors clearly delineate their role as a supervisor of midwives from their substantive role as a midwife, demonstrating how their expert knowledge of statutory supervision and clinical practice protects the public. By appointing a supervisor of midwives, the LSA ensures that support, advice and guidance are available for women and midwives 24 hours a day to ensure public protection. Supervisors have a responsibility to bring to the attention of the LSA any practice or service issues that might put at risk a midwife's ability to care for women and their babies (NMC, 2014). Effective use of the supervisory framework leads to improvements in the standard of midwifery care, thus ensuring that the care provided meets the woman's needs and that it is given in the right place and by the right person. Supervisors of midwives work with midwives to provide the best possible care for mothers and babies and there is a mutual responsibility for effective communication between midwives and supervisors of midwives.

In January 2015, following a number of critical incidents and independent reports (PHSO, 2013a, 2013b, 2013c, 2013d; Baird et al., 2014), the NMC decided to seek change to legislation governing midwives. On 16 July 2015, the Secretary of State for Health announced that the government would change the legislation as requested by the NMC. The main effect of the changes will be the removal of statutory supervision from the NMC's regulatory legislation.

The removal of statutory supervision from legislation will ensure that the NMC will bear sole responsibility for all regulatory decisions regarding midwives. However, it will not mean the end of the support, development and leadership provided by supervisors of midwives to midwives, women and their families. The Department of Health England is currently leading work to define and plan for a future for supervision outside of regulatory legislation. This work involves the four UK Chief Nursing Officers and has input from the Royal College of Midwives, the LSAMO Forum UK and the NMC.

The role of supervisors of midwives in promoting normality in labour and birth

The term 'normal birth' refers to a vaginal birth without any medical procedures that require hospital-based care, such as the use of epidural or spinal anaesthetic, induction of labour, instrumental deliveries and caesarean section. Normalizing childbirth, in contrast, is about promoting childbirth as a normal physiological process, listening to women about their birth choices and reducing unnecessary interventions.

Maternity policy in all four countries of the UK has been directed towards offering women access to midwife-led services with an explicit focus on promoting normal birth and reducing interventions (Department of Health, 2004; NHS QIS, 2009; DHSSPSNI, 2012). In England, standards are in place that require services to 'ensure that pregnant women receive high quality care throughout their pregnancy, have a *normal childbirth* wherever possible, are *involved in decisions* about what is best for them and *have choices about how and where they give birth*' (Department of Health, 2004: 9, emphasis added). In Scotland, the Keeping Childbirth Natural and Dynamic (KCND) pathway was designed to facilitate ongoing risk assessment and to ensure evidence-based care by the appropriate professional for all women accessing maternity care across Scotland: 'The ethos of the pathway is that pregnancy and childbirth are *normal physiological processes and unnecessary intervention should be avoided*' (NHS QIS, 2009: 2, emphasis added). And in Northern Ireland, 'the LSAMO, along with each of the Trust's supervisors of midwives . . . have a pivotal leadership role in the promotion of the skills of the midwife, *normalising birth, reduction of intervention rates*, and ensuring models of care, including midwife-led units and home births, are safe, sustainable and *family-centred*' (DHSSPSNI, 2012: 29, emphasis added).

In their analysis of the LSA annual reports, the NMC established that there continues to be a commitment by supervisors across the UK to promote normality in childbirth and reduce rates of intervention, thus promoting the health and well-being of women (NMC, 2012b, 2013). For example:

- In London, supervisors are promoting normal birth, including water births and vaginal birth after caesarean (VBAC), through working alongside midwives and are involved in individualized care planning with women who have chosen particular options of care that may not meet national and local recommendations (London LSA, 2013).

- In the East of England, supervisors led on a normal birth campaign that looked at reducing the number of caesarean sections that are not medically necessary, and have led and actively supported VBAC clinics. This has included the implementation of a pathway to help women achieve a VBAC (East of England LSA, 2013).

- In Scotland, supervisors are leading on the development, implementation and evaluation of a philosophy of normality in labour (South East & West of Scotland LSAs, 2013).

- And in Wales, supervisors have hosted active birth and normality workshops as part of the annual update training offered to all midwives and have been working with midwives to reduce the incidence of caesarean section (Healthcare Inspectorate Wales 2013).

For the majority of women, birth is safe and uncomplicated. However, for some women, risk factors may be present prior to pregnancy or become apparent during pregnancy that present challenges for midwifery practice and the associated supervisory support. For example, some maternity units report that as many as 50% of their pregnant population are clinically obese with a body mass index (BMI) >35, and continued high rates of smoking and drinking present particular challenges to maternity services and to the health of the women and their babies (East of England LSA, 2013; Healthcare Inspectorate Wales, 2013).

Supervisors of midwives are crucial in promoting the core role of the midwife and supporting them in adapting to the changing clinical landscape. They work collaboratively with members of the multidisciplinary team and governance teams to improve standards of care and ensure that service delivery models are safe, family-centred and evidence-based (Department of Health, 2010). An example of what can be achieved is a project in the East Midlands where two midwives, supported by a supervisor of midwives, were designated to work with pregnant women with a BMI >30. For women with a BMI between 30 and 34.9, this included brief interventions and an exercise referral. For those with a BMI of 35 and above, they were offered seven one-to-one intervention sessions with the aim of limiting weight gain during pregnancy to the 5–9 kg recommended. The outcome of the project showed reductions in the women's blood pressures and the incidence of pre-eclampsia. Other pregnancy complications were reduced by 67% and labour complications by 75% (East Midlands LSA, 2013).

Another example of supervisors helping midwives consider how they can facilitate women who are historically seen as high risk, is demonstrated in the use of low-risk technology in labour and birth (e.g. a birthing pool). This approach is supported through reviewing guidelines on Group B streptococcus and VBAC in respect of using telemetry in the pool (conversation on 7 July 2014 with L. Hicken, Supervisor of Midwives England).

An important factor that supervisors have to consider is the rising proportion of births to older women, especially as older maternal age may be associated with pre-existing ill health, low fertility, complications of pregnancy and an increased risk of adverse outcomes, including stillbirths and congenital anomalies (Jacobsson et al., 2004; ISD Scotland, 2014). In these circumstances, continuous and appropriate risk assessment with good communication between professionals and the woman is essential to achieving safe outcomes – the emphasis being on positive risk assessment not negative risk assessment based on discussion with the woman followed by good record-keeping. In Scotland, supervisors are committed to help achieve the Scottish Patient Safety Programme goals to reduce avoidable harm in women and babies by 30% by 2015. They also aim to increase the percentage of women satisfied with their experience of maternity care to >95% by 2015 by raising awareness of the programme and its initiatives with supervisees and being agents for change (Scottish Patient Safety Programme, 2013).

Practice point

Supervisors of midwives promote the normalization of childbirth by being involved in the development of strategies, guidelines and services based on evidence and not by taking risks or encouraging women to take risks.

Women's right to choose and a midwife's duty of care

Midwives are working under great pressure alongside women with increasing complexities of health needs, high levels of public expectation and rising birth rates. This provides an environment where significant support, specific development and encouragement are required for midwives to provide the high-quality care that every woman and their family deserve. Supervisors of midwives are increasingly called upon to offer support to both women and midwives in difficult situations, especially in relation to the complexity of births.

Through the supervisory framework, LSAs work collaboratively with supervisors of midwives, approved education institutions (AEIs) and employers to ensure all midwives continue to have the necessary skills to deliver safe and effective care. This is evident through local post-registration education and training for midwives, including regular skills and drills practice, high-dependency midwifery care and participation in pre-registration midwifery programmes to promote caring for women with complicated and high-risk pregnancies (NMC, 2013).

Right to choose

Pregnant women are entitled to make autonomous decisions in the same way as anyone else. Their decisions must be respected, regardless of whether health professionals agree with them. The principle of autonomy creates a legal requirement to obtain a woman's consent whenever treatment is offered. Exceptions to this occur when either the woman does not have the capacity to make her own decisions or in an emergency when she cannot consent because of her physical condition. For consent to be valid, the woman must be informed about the proposed treatment/care provision and she should not be put under any undue pressure by healthcare professionals or family members into receiving the treatment/care (NHS Choices, 2014).

Treatment and/or care provided in the absence of a woman's consent constitutes the crime of battery, a civil wrong of trespass to the person and violates Article 8 of the European Convention of Human Rights (ECHR/Council of Europe, undated). Any serious harm that occurs as a result of treatment/care in the absence of consent will also breach Article 3 of the European Convention of Human Rights (undated) prohibiting inhuman and degrading treatment. The NMC and the General Medical Council (GMC) produce guidance on consent, explaining in detail what information midwives and doctors are expected to provide as well as how consent should be recorded. The Royal College of Obstetricians and Gynaecologists (RCOG) also provides advice on consent, and on specific procedures and the risks associated with those procedures, including caesarean section and operative vaginal birth (see Further reading to access all of the above resources).

Information provided to a woman to enable her to make an informed decision should cover any significant risks, alternative treatments/care available and the risks of doing nothing. Although the law does not require that doctors and midwives provide women with all the information within their knowledge, they must provide enough information so that the general nature and purpose of the treatment are properly understood. Failure to provide appropriate information may leave the healthcare professional open to a successful claim of negligence where the woman suffers harm as a result of the treatment/care provided. If a woman asks specific questions, it is good practice for a healthcare professional to give full, honest and objective answers. The woman decides whether to accept any of the options on offer and, if so, which one. She also has the right to accept or refuse an option for a reason that may seem irrational to the health professional, or for no reason at all. According to Green et al. (2003), what is important to women in labour is the quality of the interactions that they have with their caregivers, especially being treated as an individual and with respect. Feeling in control of what professionals are doing is the most important variable for women but having choices is also important. A sense of control is critical to subsequent psychological wellbeing.

While women have experienced an increase in alternative forms of birthing options in midwifery-led units, including personalized birthing centres, a reduction in home births has been noted. It is often women with complex pregnancies and against medical advice who are increasingly wishing to give birth at home despite these alternative options.

Case 4.1: Emma

Emma was a 43-year-old gravida 3. In her first labour, Emma suffered from high blood pressure and was admitted to the high dependency area on the labour suite. She was put on a cardiotocograph (CTG), kept in bed, and not allowed to get up to mobilize as the fetal heart needed to be monitored effectively. Labour did not progress and Emma had a caesarean section. She said: 'I didn't feel involved with the whole birth – it was just something that was passively happening to me.' The repercussion of this experience was that Emma was diagnosed as having postnatal depression but was subsequently informed that she was actually suffering from post-traumatic stress disorder.

With her second pregnancy, Emma decided to have a VBAC at home. The supervisor of midwives put in place a birth plan for Emma and everyone was aware of this. For the first time, Emma felt that people listened to her – she said that the supervisor of midwives was the key to this approach and that midwives looked to the supervisor for direction and even the obstetrician who was in charge of her case listened to the supervisor's advice.

Emma went on to have her baby at home. She said that achieving a vaginal birth at home meant she was able to trust her body and that the stress from her first delivery, of feeling a failure, went away. She said: 'When I was giving birth I realized that I did know what to do, that my body knew what to do . . . I couldn't have asked for a better experience.'

Practice point

Women will be more willing to engage with supervisors/midwives if approached early in pregnancy rather than in the later stages of pregnancy when they feel most vulnerable.

Midwives' duty of care

Duty of care is the obligation that healthcare professionals have towards those in their care; it is not something that can be ignored or put aside. For a midwife, duty of care is the requirement that she acts in a way that ensures that the needs of the woman and her baby are the primary focus of her practice. This is achieved by working in partnership with the woman and her family providing safe, responsive care in an environment that meets the woman's physical and emotional needs throughout childbirth and is consistent with high standards of practice.

The rules and standards for midwives (NMC, 2012b) define a midwife's obligations and scope of practice (Box 4.2) while the Code of Conduct (NMC, 2008) underpins professional practice (Box 4.3). However, on occasions a midwife may find herself in a situation where her duty of care is in conflict with a woman's birth plan and her employer's expectations, such as when a woman requests a pathway of care that falls outside national and local recommendations. One of the biggest challenges for midwives is when women who are deemed as having complex needs or who are 'high risk' choose a 'low-risk' approach to their labour and birth – for example, deciding on a home birth against medical advice or refusing all care offered, in effect 'free birthing'. However, not all women who want no or minimal intervention choose to give birth at home; many will choose to use the services offered at the maternity unit but refuse interventions such as induction of labour. In these professional encounters with women, midwives cannot rely solely on standards, codes, protocols and practice guidelines; they also have to use their experience and professional judgement. Complex situations can arise when there is an apparent conflict between the woman's choice, her safety and that of her unborn baby. This particular dilemma is a difficult one for midwives, and it is very important that a considered and measured approach is worked through with the woman and her family on case-by-case basis; it is important to discuss any health issues, if they develop, with the woman.

Box 4.2: Rule 5 – Scope of practice

Rule 5:1   You must be capable of meeting the competencies and essential skills clusters set out in standard 17 of the *Standards for pre-registration midwifery education (2009)* that are within your scope of practice.

Rule 5:2   You must make sure the needs of the woman and her baby are the primary focus of your practice and you should work in partnership with the woman and her family, providing safe, responsive, compassionate care in an appropriate environment to facilitate her physical and emotional care throughout childbirth.

Rule 5:3   Except in an emergency, you must not provide care, or undertake any treatment, that you have not been trained to give.

Rule 5:4   In an emergency, or where a deviation from the norm, which is outside of your current sphere of practice, becomes apparent in a woman or baby during childbirth, you must call such health or social care professionals as may reasonably be expected to have the necessary skills and experience to assist you in the provision of care.

Source: NMC (2012b).

Box 4.3: The Code – Standards of conduct, performance and ethics for nurses and midwives: summary of relevant principles

The people in your care must be able to trust you with their health and wellbeing

To justify that trust, you must: *make the care of people your first concern, treating them as individuals and respecting their dignity*

Treat people as individuals
Collaborate with those in your care
Ensure you gain consent

Work with others to protect and promote the health and wellbeing of those in your care, their families and carers, and the wider community

Share information with your colleagues
Work effectively as part of a team
Manage risk

Provide a high standard of practice and care at all times

Use the best available evidence
Keep your skills and knowledge up to date
Keep clear and accurate records

Be open and honest, act with integrity and uphold the reputation of your profession

Act with integrity

Source: NMC (2008).

The supervisor of midwives can provide guidance and support to the midwife to ensure she understands her duty of care to the woman and her employer and what she can do to assist the woman in achieving her birth plan while maintaining professional standards. The supervisor will also support midwives in best practice if others are advocating an approach to care that is not supported by the evidence (LSAMO Forum UK, 2009). Midwives should feel able to ask another midwife or a supervisor for advice and guidance when a woman's labour is not going to plan – this is a strength, not a weakness.

Practice point

'. . . midwives must at all times and under all circumstances act in accordance with professional obligations and judgement and not do something that is inconsistent with or contrary to professional training, integrity or which could be justified at a later date as consistent with good practice and sound professional judgement'. (Flaxman Partners, 2011: 53)

Case 4.2: Anne

Anne, aged 43, was a schoolteacher who was pregnant with her first child. At booking, Anne informed her midwife that she wanted to have a home birth. The midwife informed Anne that local policy dictated that 'elderly' primiparous women had to deliver in the obstetric unit, and so she would not be allowed to deliver at home. Anne refused to discuss her plan with the midwife and demanded to see a senior midwife. An arrangement was made for Anne to meet with a supervisor of midwives.

At the meeting with the supervisor, Anne stated that she would be having a home birth and that she would not allow the midwives to attend; although she would agree to them being in her house during her labour and birth, she would not allow them to examine her. Anne clearly stated that if the midwives tried to examine her to assess her or her baby's wellbeing, she would sue. By carefully listening to Anne and the reasons for her request, the supervisor established that Anne had a phobia about hospitals and did not trust health professionals in general, the result of an experience she had when she was a teenager. The supervisor advised Anne about her rights and made sure she was aware of all the choices available to her. Following this discussion, Anne decided that she still wanted a home birth and still did not want any midwives to examine her during labour and birth.

The supervisor of midwives then met with the midwives and ensured that they were aware of Anne's right to make a decision about her place of birth even though they thought that she would be safer delivering in the obstetric unit. The importance of building a trusting relationship with Anne was emphasized, as was the importance of ensuring Anne was enabled to make informed decisions. The supervisor maintained contact with Anne throughout her pregnancy and gave continuing support to the midwives. This approach was successful – the midwives built a trusting relationship with Anne to the point that she agreed they could attend during her labour and birth at home and could examine her to assess her and her baby's wellbeing.

Anne laboured at home with her midwives present. Unfortunately, the labour did not progress and a fetal tachycardia developed. Following a full discussion with the midwives, Anne agreed to transfer to the obstetric unit where an obstetrician reviewed her and an emergency caesarean section was performed. Despite having a caesarean section, Anne informed the supervisor of midwives that she was not disappointed that her plan to have a home birth had not been achieved; this, she said, was because she had been listened to and given control over decisions about her care.

Practice point

Listen to the woman to facilitate understanding of what she actually wants and why she wants to go in that direction – it's understanding 'why' that is important.

Effective communication

To enable women to make informed choices about their care pathway, they need to have clear unambiguous information about their pregnancy, including any actual or perceived risks and the services available to them. Midwives have a responsibility to provide evidence-based, up-to-date information and give advice to women accessing maternity care. Many maternity units have developed leaflets to inform women of their choices, although O'Cathain et al. (2002: 643) have established that 'in everyday practice, evidence based leaflets were not effective in promoting informed choice in women using maternity services'. For this reason, it is important that good communication between the midwife and the woman is maintained throughout the pregnancy. The woman should be encouraged to prepare a birth plan that includes addressing any concerns or fears.

When writing a birth plan with a woman, a midwife should make notes before putting the plan in writing and sending it back to the woman to read and amend as required. It is important that the woman sees, understands and agrees with what has been written before it is cascaded to the wider team (conversation on 7 July 2014 with L. Hicken, Supervisor of Midwives). It is essential to build a good rapport with the woman to establish a trusting relationship.

Midwives should discuss the risks and benefits without using strong emotive language, such as 'your baby might die if you chose that path'. A written record must be made of the discussion that has taken place between the woman and the midwife. This documentation in the woman's maternity record should demonstrate that the woman has been fully informed of the risks and benefits identified in relation to her care, the choices available and any recommendations that have been made to her, and that she understands this information. Communication with the whole of the multidisciplinary team will also facilitate support for all involved (NMC, 2009).

It is important to remember, however, that it is not just women who choose a home birth who are informed of risk – women who choose a hospital birth should also be informed of the risks and benefits of their chosen care pathway.

Women have a responsibility to acknowledge the information and advice they have been given even if they choose not to engage with such advice. Women also need to understand that although midwives are highly skilled, there are limitations to their scope of practice (conversation on 11 July 2014 with J. Horn, Supervisor of Midwives). Supervisors of midwives are well placed to provide support and advice to midwives and women in these complex circumstances.

When a woman who is classified as 'high risk' or has a 'complex pregnancy' requests a home birth, a supervisor may see her in her own home, as this promotes privacy and confidentiality and any interruptions are of the woman's making rather than of the supervisor of midwives (conversation on 7 July 2014 with L. Hicken, Supervisor of Midwives). This meeting provides an opportunity to unpick the woman's particular issues and understand what it is she wants and why she wants it. The supervisor is then in a better position to discuss options with the woman and enable her to make an informed choice.

Midwives should feel able to ask another midwife or supervisor for advice and guidance when a woman's labour is not going to plan – this should be seen as a strength, not a weakness. It is also important to discuss issues as they develop with the woman; this gives the woman options, keeps the dialogue open, and demonstrates that the midwife values her views and thoughts and sees her as an individual.

Practice point

Communication with the woman and her family should be respectful and seek to maintain an open dialogue. Over-emphasis and repetition of risks once understood by the woman may be unhelpful and create alienation.

Case 4.3: Lorna

Lorna was a 38-year-old gravida 4 – para 3+1. Her first pregnancy was ectopic and resulted in the removal of a fallopian tube. She also suffered from endometriosis. In 2010, Lorna conceived again. However, from 9 weeks gestation she experienced persistent vaginal bleeding. Lorna knew something was wrong but was just told by midwives and obstetricians that some people 'bleed during pregnancy'. At 22 weeks gestation, Lorna was admitted to the obstetric unit as the bleeding became heavy and following a scan was informed that there was no liquor around the baby. She was also informed that she would have to have a caesarean section because the baby was small and in a breech presentation; there was no discussion regarding her birth choices. At 26+ weeks, Lorna was transferred to another obstetric unit because there were no neonatal cots available where she currently was. Here, birth choices were discussed with her and she was advised that a caesarean section might not be appropriate, especially in respect of the size of the baby and any future pregnancies. Lorna felt more informed and involved in her care: 'we were told what we were dealing with', she sais. Unfortunately, following a scan at 27 weeks gestation, it was established that the baby had died following a placental abruption.

Following these events, Lorna was not offered a debriefing although she was offered a copy of her maternity notes. Importantly, Lorna was not made aware of the support available to her through the statutory supervision of midwives; it is apparent that she would have benefited from having all her care options explained to her and having an advocate to speak on her behalf.

In a subsequent pregnancy, Lorna was told she could have whatever she wanted in relation to her labour and birth: she said, 'we made the choices'. Because she was fully involved in all decisions, she felt much more positive about this preg nancy than she had felt previously. Initially, she wanted a caesarean section but following discussion agreed to be induced at 38 weeks gestation. However, this was a much better experience, although she was confined to bed during labour by the attending midwife, as the fetal heart had to be continuously monitored.

By her third labour, Lorna was supported to be mobile and enabled to do things her way. She said; 'although I was in pain, all I can remember is laughing . . . I was empowered . . . this birth I could do again today . . . I have fabulous memories'. This positive experience was made possible because the midwives listened to her and respected her wishes.

Practice point

Ensure women are fully informed of the options of care available to them, thereby ensuring genuine informed, shared decision-making.

Conclusion

Appropriate systems that are transparent and clear to both midwives and women are vital for managing potential problems and preventing them from escalating into a more urgent situation. Supervisors of midwives have a vital role to play here in offering guidance and support to women about any aspect of their midwifery care, including providing advice about the various options of care available, advocating for the right of women to make informed choices about their care, and monitoring the ability and behaviour of midwives to ensure that they meet the standards set by the NMC (NMC, 2012a, 2014). With good planning, strong communication and sound protocols in place, all parties will be enabled to make appropriate and reasonable decisions.

Acknowledgements

Thanks to L. Hicken, Supervisor of Midwives, Southmead Hospital, Westbury-on-Trym, North Bristol NHS Trust, and J. Horn, Supervisor of Midwives, Royal Bournemouth and Christchurch Hospitals NHS Foundation Trust for sharing with me their experiences of supporting women with challenging or complex pregnancies when they request no or little intervention in their labours and births.

Further reading

General Medical Council (GMC). The GMC produces guidance on consent explaining in detail what information doctors are expected to provide, as well as how consent should be recorded [http://www.gmc-uk.org/guidance/ethical_guidance/consent_guidance_index.asp].

LSAMO Forum UK. Information on the statutory supervision of midwives is available through the LSAMO Forum UK website [http://www.lsamoforumuk.scot.nhs.uk/]

Nursing and Midwifery Council (NMC). The NMC produces guidance on consent explaining in detail what information nurses and midwives are expected to provide, as well as how consent should be recorded [http://www.nmc-uk.org/Nurses-and-midwives/Regulation-in-practice/Regulation-in-Practice-Topics/consent].

Royal College of Midwives (RCM). The RCM has a website on promoting normal birth, including its ten top tips and birthing positions [http://www.rcmnormalbirth.org.uk].

Royal College of Obstetricians and Gynaecologists (RCOG). The College provides advice on consent, and on specific procedures and the risks associated with those procedures, including caesarean section and operative vaginal birth [https://www.rcog.org.uk/en/guidelines-research-services/guidelines/?q=&subject=&type=Consent+Advice&orderby=title].

References

Bacon, L. (2011) What does the future hold for the role of the Local Supervising Authority?, *British Journal of Midwifery*, 19 (7): 439–42.

Baird, B., Murray, R., Seale, B., Foot, C. and Perry, C. (2014) *Midwifery Regulation in the United Kingdom*. London: King's Fund [http://www.nmc.org.uk/globalassets/sitedocuments/councilpapersanddocuments/council-2015/kings-fund-review.pdf].

Department of Health (2004) *National Service Framework for Children, Young People and Maternity Services*. London: DH Publications [https://www.gov.uk/government/uploads/system/uploads/attachment_data/file/199952/National_Service_Framework_for_Children_Young_People_and_Maternity_Services_-_Core_Standards.pdf; accessed 5 May 2014].

Department of Health (2010) *Midwifery 2020: Delivering expectations.* London: Department of Health [https://www.gov.uk/government/publications/midwifery-2020-delivering-expectations; accessed 7 June 2014].
Department of Health, Social Services and Public Safety: Northern Ireland (DHSSPSNI) (2012) *A Strategy for Maternity Care in Northern Ireland 2012–2018* [https://www.dhsspsni.gov.uk/publications/strategy-maternity-care-northern-ireland-2012-2018; accessed 15 October 2014].
East Midlands LSA (2013) *Annual Report to the Nursing and Midwifery Council 1 April 2012–31 March 2013* [https://www.nmc.org.uk/standards/what-to-expect-from-a-nurse-or-midwife/how-midwives-are-regulated/lsa-reports/; accessed 3 July 2014].
East of England LSA (2013) *Annual Report to the Nursing and Midwifery Council 1 April 2012–31 March 2013* [https://www.nmc.org.uk/standards/what-to-expect-from-a-nurse-or-midwife/how-midwives-are-regulated/lsa-reports/; accessed 3 July 2014].
European Court of Human Rights/Council of Europe (undated) *European Convention of Human Rights* [http://www.echr.coe.int/Documents/Convention_ENG.pdf; accessed 13 October 2014].
Flaxman Partners (2011) *The Feasibility and Insurability of Independent Midwifery in England.* London: Nursing and Midwifery Council [http://www.nmc-uk.org/Documents/Midwifery-Reports/Feasibility-and-Insurability-of-Independent-Midwifery-in-England_September-2011.pdf; accessed 20 June 2014].
Green, J., Baston, H., Easton, S. and McCormick, F. (2003) *Greater Expectations? Summary report.* Leeds: Mother and Infant Research Unit, University of Leeds.
Healthcare Inspectorate Wales (2013) *Annual Report to the Nursing and Midwifery Council 1st April 2012–31st March 2013* [http://www.nmc-uk.org/Nurses-and-midwives/Midwifery-New/NMC-LSA-reports/Wales-LSA-Report; accessed 13 October 2014].
Horton, R. (2008) What does a National Health Service mean in the 21st century?, *Lancet*, 371 (9631): 2213–18.
Information Services Division (ISD) Scotland (2014) *Maternity and Births* [http://www.isdscotland.org/Health-Topics/Maternity-and-births/index.asp?Co=Y; accessed 7 November 2014].
Jacobsson, B., Ladfors, L. and Milsom, I. (2004) Advanced maternal age and adverse perinatal outcome, *Obstetrics and Gynecology*, 104 (4): 727–33.
London LSA (2013) *Annual Report to the Nursing and Midwifery Council 1st April 2012–31st March 2013* [https://www.nmc.org.uk/standards/what-to-expect-from-a-nurse-or-midwife/how-midwives-are-regulated/lsa-reports/; accessed 3 July 2014].
LSAMO Forum UK (2009) *Modern Supervision in Action: A Practical Guide for Midwives* [http://www.lsamoforumuk.scot.nhs.uk/midwives.aspx; accessed 13 July 2014].
Midwives Act, 1902 [2 Edw. 7. c. 17].
Midwives (Ireland) Act 1918 [7 & 8 Geo. 5 c. 56].
Midwives (Scotland) Act, 1915 [5 & 6 Geo. 5. c. 91].
NHS Choices (2014) *Consent to Treatment* [http://www.nhs.uk/conditions/Consent-to-treatment/Pages/Introduction.aspx; accessed 7 November 2014].
NHS Quality Improvement Scotland (NHS QIS) (2009) *Keeping Childbirth Natural and Dynamic: Pathways for maternity care* [http://www.healthcareimprovementscotland.org/our_work/reproductive,_maternal_child/programme_resources/keeping_childbirth_natural.aspx; accessed 13 October 2014].
Nursing and Midwifery Council (NMC) (2008) *The Code: Standards of conduct, performance and ethics for nurses and midwives.* London: NMC [http://www.nmc-uk.org/Publications/Standards; accessed 7 November 2014].

Nursing and Midwifery Council (NMC) (2009) *Record Keeping: Guidance for nurses and midwives*. London: NMC [http://www.nmc-uk.org/Publications/Guidance; accessed 7 November 2014].

Nursing and Midwifery Council (NMC) (2012a) *Supervisors of Midwives: How they can help you*. London: NMC [http://www.nmc-uk.org/Publications/Information-for-the-public; accessed 13 October 2014].

Nursing and Midwifery Council (NMC) (2012b) *Midwives' Rules and Standards*. London: NMC [http://www.nmc-uk.org/Publications/Standards; accessed 7 November 2014].

Nursing and Midwifery Council (NMC) (2013) *Supervision, Support and Safety: Report of the quality assurance of the local supervising authorities 2012–2013*. London: NMC [http://www.nmc-uk.org/Publications/Midwifery-Supervision; accessed 13 October 2014].

Nursing and Midwifery Council (NMC) (2014) *Standards for the Preparation of Supervisors of Midwives*. London: NMC [http://www.nmc-uk.org/Publications/Standards; accessed 13 October 2014].

O'Cathain, A., Walters, S.J., Nicholl, J.P., Thomas, K.J. and Kirkham, M. (2002) Use of evidence based leaflets to promote informed choice in maternity care: randomised controlled trial in everyday practice, *British Medical Journal*, 324: 643–6.

Parliamentary and Health Services Ombudsman (PHSO) (2013a) *Midwifery Supervision and Regulation: A report by the Health Service Ombudsman of an investigation into a complaint from Mr L about the North West Strategic Health Authority* [http://www.ombudsman.org.uk/__data/assets/pdf_file/0019/23383/NWSHA-MR-L-Report.pdf].

Parliamentary and Health Services Ombudsman (PHSO) (2013b) *Midwifery Supervision and Regulation: A report by the Health Service Ombudsman of an investigation into a complaint from Mr M about the North West Strategic Health Authority* [http://www.ombudsman.org.uk/__data/assets/pdf_file/0004/23494/NWSHA-MR-M-Report-2.pdf].

Parliamentary and Health Services Ombudsman (PHSO) (2013c) *Midwifery Supervision and Regulation: A report by the Health Service Ombudsman of an investigation into a complaint from Ms Q and Mr R about the North West Strategic Health Authority* [http://www.ombudsman.org.uk/__data/assets/pdf_file/0009/23499/NWSHA-MS-Q-and-MR-R-Report.pdf].

Parliamentary and Health Services Ombudsman (PHSO) (2013d) *Midwifery Supervision and Regulation: Recommendations for change* [http://www.ombudsman.org.uk/__data/assets/pdf_file/0003/23484/Midwifery-supervision-and-regulation_-recommendations-for-change.pdf].

Read, J. and Wallace, V. (2014) Supervision in action: an introduction, *British Journal of Midwifery*, 22 (3): 59–62.

Scottish Patient Safety Programme (2013) Maternity & Children Quality Improvement Collaborative (MCQIC) [http://www.scottishpatientsafetyprogramme.scot.nhs.uk/programmes/mcqic; accessed 15 October 2014].

South East & West of Scotland LSAs (2013) *Annual Report to the Nursing and Midwifery Council April 2012–March 2013* [https://www.nmc.org.uk/standards/what-to-expect-from-a-nurse-or-midwife/how-midwives-are-regulated/lsa-reports/; accessed 3 July 2014].

The Nursing and Midwifery Order 2001 (SI: 2002 /253) [http://www.legislation.gov.uk/uksi/2002/253/made; accessed 7 November 2014].

United Nations (1948) *Universal Declaration of Human Rights* [http://www.un.org/en/documents/udhr/index.shtml; accessed 17 June 2014].

United Nations (2000) *Substantive Issues Arising in the Implementation of the International Covenant on Economic, Social and Cultural Rights. General comment no 14. The right to the highest attainable standard of health (Article 12 of the International Covenant on Economic, Social and Cultural Rights)* [http://data.unaids.org/publications/external-documents/ecosoc_cescr-gc14_en.pdf; accessed 17 June 2014].

United Nations General Assembly (1966) *International Covenant on Economic, Social and Cultural Rights*, 16 December 1966, United Nations, Treaty Series, Vol. 993, p. 3 [http://www.refworld.org/docid/3ae6b36c0.html; accessed 12 August 2014].

5

Fear of childbirth: the impact of tocophobia (including post-traumatic stress disorder) on normal birth

Clare Gribbin

Introduction

This chapter is intended to be thought-provoking and challenging as well as informative. It concentrates on two separate but overlapping subjects in relation to childbirth: tocophobia and post-traumatic stress disorder (PTSD). An understanding of how these two are distinct and how they relate is essential when considering how fear of childbirth impacts on normal birth and how as professionals we can limit its impact on the women we serve. Anonymized case illustrations will outline some of the challenges and issues in care. The intention is to outline the meaning and context for the terms and diagnoses used, thus further developing understanding, care and management. The ultimate goal is to play our part in enabling women to achieve positive experiences of childbirth.

Challenges in defining 'fear of childbirth', 'tocophobia' and 'normal birth'

The word 'tocophobia' originates from the Greek 'tokos', which means childbirth and 'phobos', which means fear. There are a variety of definitions in circulation that help to give us an understanding of its application and use. The first example below is from *Collins Dictionary* (2016) while the remaining four examples are collated from *Encyclo* (2016), an English online encyclopaedia:

*   'An abnormal fear of giving birth or becoming pregnant' (*Collins Dictionary*, 2016);
*   'An abnormal and persistent fear of childbirth. A phobia is an unreasonable fear that can cause avoidance and panic. Phobias are a relatively common type of anxiety disorder';
*   'an irrational fear of childbirth';
*   'an excessive fear of childbirth';
*   'a morbid dread of childbirth' (*Encyclo*, 2016).

It is reasonable to conclude from the above that a precise definition is challenging to find. Arguably, the first definition is the most helpful, as it explicitly encompasses women at all stages including pre-pregnancy. Implicit in this definition is also the concept that, for some women, being pregnant can be a 'fearful' experience and that some level of fear is normal and to be expected. It is only when there is 'abnormal fear' that a diagnosis of tocophobia can be made.

The phrase 'normal birth' opens up a myriad of thoughts and images, different for each individual and not unified across healthcare professionals. What is meant by the term 'normal birth' and do all practitioners have the same understanding? Do we mean unassisted vaginal birth? (See Chapter 1 for definitions of 'normal birth'.) If so, by implication does this mean that all other methods of birth are somehow abnormal?

There are cultural, social and psychological implications of the precise words we use. Terminology is a critical factor for many women. For example, current trends lead professionals to use the term 'birthed', which is seen to be more acceptable than 'delivered', which has more paternalistic connotations. Defining what is meant in context is essential in ensuring that everyone starts with the same level of understanding. Many readers of this book may have started with different interpretations of the words in the title: 'Normalizing challenging or complex childbirth'. Some may think that by the term 'normalizing', what is meant is 'making it acceptable to give birth with assistance', while others may interpret the title as meaning 'achieving a vaginal birth with little or no intervention'. My own favoured interpretation (and that of the authors of other chapters) is to 'humanize the birthing process even in cases where intervention is necessary'.

The challenge for professionals is to aspire to all meanings simultaneously – acceptance for the operative (assisted birth) where needed while at the same time increasing the ability to facilitate more spontaneous vaginal births in all women, including those in the high-risk groups. Professionals should work together to focus on each individual woman, her psychological wellbeing, personal experience, self-esteem and safety. The environment and provision of one-to-one care should be the same for everyone, irrespective of the journey to or precise mode of birthing. In units where this is achieved, I believe that the feeling of 'failure' or 'abnormality' that some women experience in our care who do need assistance is reduced. It also prevents unnecessary interventions in both low- and high-risk women.

An interesting gender assumption is usually made in most writing exploring fear of childbirth and tocophobia. The assumption is that tocophobia applies solely to women. However, men can also experience tocophobia, although there is limited literature on the topic. In my personal practice, I have seen couples where the male partner has been affected by tocophobia. By searching the internet for 'tocophobia in men', it is possible to access a variety of information, although to my knowledge there has been no high-quality research. Key issues rest with challenges in definition and the understandable difficulty for individuals to acknowledge, disclose or discuss their fears.

Throughout this chapter, midwives and obstetricians are referred to as 'clinicians' although, where needed, the title midwife or obstetrician will be used to distinguish between the two.

Tocophobia

Tocophobia in the context of phobia

Phobias are a part of the classification anxiety disorders (APA, 2013, previously APA, 2000). Approximately 10 million people in the UK have a phobia. They are the most common type of anxiety disorder and can affect anyone. A phobia can be defined as an overwhelming and debilitating fear of an object, place, situation, feeling or animal. Contact, thoughts or associations with the source of the phobia can produce the well-known characteristic symptoms of anxiety. These may include dizziness, nausea, sweating, palpitations, a shortness of breath, shaking, vomiting, and so on. There is a range of severity of expression in terms of symptoms and frequency. Phobias do not have a single cause. Box 5.1 highlights how the causes of tocophobia relate to the three common associations of general phobias.

Box 5.1: The three common associations of general phobias

A phobia may be associated with a particular incident or trauma. Tocophobia may stem from a negative experience in adolescence or childhood, such as seeing or hearing about a birth (either real or depicted) with no support or explanation. It may relate to a previous difficult birth experience with a negative outcome. Examples include perceived threat to life of mother or baby, stillbirth or neonatal admission. Tocophobia may also result from a normal birth where communication was poor or expectations unfulfilled (postnatal PTSD or depression may have resulted).

A phobia may be a learned response from someone else. Tocophobia may be a learned response from a mother or relative passing on their negative and fearful views of childbirth. This could be passed on to a daughter or a son.

A phobia may have a genetic component, as some people are more predisposed to anxiety than others (Fyer et al., 1990; Kendler et al., 1999). The specific cause in these situations may remain unknown. According to Skre et al. (2000), evidence for genetic transmission is variable across phobia types and is highest for blood-injection-injury phobias and lowest for natural environment and situational phobias. This means that there is less evidence for a genetic basis to tocophobia than other phobia types.

Phobias are well documented in the literature (e.g. Curtis et al., 1998; NICE, 2009, 2011a; McCabe et al., 2010). Simple phobias tend to start in childhood and adolescence and are often more straightforward to manage, partly because they become less severe with age. More complex phobias often present in adulthood, are commonly situational and can be more challenging to manage.

Most people with a phobia are fully aware of it and are able to manage the phobia without the help of others. Often this involves avoidance of the trigger.

Those with significant symptoms that disrupt wellbeing and daily living may require intervention from professionals. Most phobias can be successfully treated and cured. Simple phobias can be treated using desensitization techniques, while complex phobias can be treated with talking therapies such as counselling, psychotherapy or cognitive behavioural therapy. Medications such as beta-blockers or antidepressants can be used to treat the anxiety symptoms but not the underlying phobia.

Tocophobia could be described as similar to other phobias in most regards. However, there are some important differences. Some women may not know that they have tocophobia until they are pregnant because the fear does not increase to a phobic level until this time (Wijma, 2003). Unlike other phobias that usually can be controlled by avoidance, this is not an option for the tocophobic pregnant woman. The only real possibility of avoidance once pregnant would be termination of pregnancy. Once pregnant, the tocophobic woman feels she cannot avoid what she most fears: she is out of control (Hofberg and Brockington, 2000). In reality, a number of women go ahead with termination of pregnancy, not because they don't want a baby but because their fear of pregnancy or childbirth is so great that they action the avoidance behaviour and seek termination. Others choose to avoid pregnancy altogether or adopt children as a method of avoidance of childbirth (Hofberg and Ward, 2003).

Primary and secondary tocophobia

Tocophobia can be categorized into primary and secondary tocophobia, as described by Hofberg and Ward (2003). Primary tocophobia can occur at any stage of a woman's reproductive life. The onset can be as early as adolescence or may not become apparent until there is a real possibility of pregnancy. For some women, the fear of pregnancy or birth can be so great that they use several methods of contraception simultaneously and never seek help to overcome their fear despite their desire to have children. A small subset of women with tocophobia will have severe vaginismus, failing to consummate their relationship with their partner due to a desire to prevent even the possibility of pregnancy. They may present in other settings with anxiety symptoms or to termination services (Hofberg and Ward, 2003). Some may present in pregnancy to maternity services aware that they need additional support through pregnancy and birth.

Hofberg and Ward (2003) describe secondary tocophobia as that following a previous traumatic and precipitating event. Most commonly this is a previous traumatic birth but may follow sexual issues, medical examinations, assault or previous PTSD unrelated to birth. Secondary tocophobia may present postnatally when there is no immediate desire for or threat of a pregnancy in the near future.

Of those women who are able to overcome tocophobia to the extent that they can get pregnant, some do not disclose their fear while others may request elective caesarean section. Others may present with behavioural, emotional or physical symptoms that are much more subtle and difficult to categorize. Midwives and obstetricians should be alert for symptoms such as sleeplessness, anxiety symptoms, unexpected crying and sometimes aggressive or defensive requests that may represent the signs and symptoms of tocophobia. However, tocophobia should be considered as a potential underlying cause alongside other diagnoses, including domestic abuse, physical illness, or a personality or behavioural disorder. The evidence to date shows that primiparous women suffer from tocophobia more frequently than multiparous women (Hofberg and Ward, 2003).

Some women with a known or disclosed tocophobia are referred directly to obstetric services by general practitioners, psychiatrists, midwives or other healthcare professionals. The challenge for midwives and obstetricians is that women who have not previously been diagnosed with tocophobia do not come with a label. Even those with a known diagnosis may choose not to disclose it, and the referring healthcare professional may remain unaware of the symptoms, issues and risks throughout pregnancy and into the postpartum period. It is essential that our maternity assessment processes pick up the clues and ask the right questions in the right way. Only if this occurs can health professionals influence birth outcomes, including a reduction in anxiety.

According to the literature, between 1% and 10% of pregnant women have an intense, complex and multifaceted fear of childbirth. (Clearly, this excludes the group who have avoided pregnancy altogether.) A study of 8000 women in 2002 showed that 1 in 20 women were affected by an intense fear of childbirth. Fear for the baby's health was experienced by approximately 50% of the sample and 40% had a fear of pain (Geissbuehel and Eberhand, 2002). Obtaining accurate data among these different groups is extremely difficult. This in part explains the paucity of good research. Women who have tocophobia and do not receive counselling have been shown to have a very negative subsequent experience of childbirth (Waldenström et al., 2006).

Case 5.1: Susan

Summary of history
Susan was a 32-year-old primigravida who presented to an obstetric colleague requesting caesarean section. She was unable to explain why, other than that she had had a previous 'bad' experience in childhood that she did not wish to discuss. She was referred to the birth choices clinic for an opinion.

She presented as a very calm, open and confident person. She attended alone. She began to explain her request for caesarean section as to do with the 'trauma' she had suffered.

Susan had lived in a rural setting and her parents were farmers. At the age of 12 she had been playing outside with her three brothers. They had rigged up a long, thin beam of wood. As she traversed it she slipped and fell, straddling it. She was in significant pain but hobbled home. She lay on the settee and after several hours the pain became significantly worse. Her mother called the GP who attended two hours later. She recalled being examined on the downstairs sofa, as it was too uncomfortable to move her. She became tearful as she described her exposure in such a public place in the family home. She explained that although no other family members apart from her mother were present, she felt exposed and embarrassed. The GP reassured them that she should rest and take some regular painkillers.

Four hours later Susan was in such pain, looking pale and unwell that her mother phoned for an ambulance. She was taken to the local hospital 20 miles away. On arrival, she described her ordeal as 'many people' coming to look at her 'down below'. She had a large vaginal haematoma at least the size of a grapefruit. She described being rushed to the operating theatre in what felt like alarming circumstances with 'everything happening at once'. She required a transfusion of four units of blood.

Susan broke down in tears as she described the 18 days she had remained in hospital following the surgery. The large cavity of the haematoma in her vagina needed the pack to be changed regularly. This was extremely painful and caused her immense embarrassment and humiliation each time it needed to be done. She explained that some nurses were wonderful in their care and understanding but that others had made her feel like a piece of dead meat with little regard for her privacy or feelings.

She made a full recovery but was absent from school for six weeks, which had its own impact. Once sexually active as an adult, this had been initially diffi-cult but that there were no remaining sexual issues at the time of presentation.

Summary of counselling assessment and birth plan
It is not difficult to imagine the reason why this woman requested an elective caesarean section. However, it was important to explore her specific fears and reasons for requesting caesarean without jumping to erroneous conclusions. Susan was specifically worried about losing blood vaginally and the flashbacks this might result in. It was important that she fully understood that a caesarean section would not prevent vaginal blood loss. She was also pleased to discuss and understand the number of people who would be in the operating theatre, as this was not something she had considered. She had a clear diagnosis of toco-phobia with all the characteristic symptoms that had begun and increased since becoming pregnant.

At the end of the discussion, Susan was open-minded about the possibility of a vaginal birth. As part of the consultation it was important to assess the vaginal tissues in view of the previous large haematoma and also her psycholog-ical response to her vagina. Given time and privacy, she coped very well with a vaginal examination. However, there was significant scar tissue on the right lat-eral wall of the vagina. This had lost its elasticity and was significantly fibrosed, although not specifically tender. An added concern was this area of tissue would not stretch to allow delivery of the head and would represent a tissue trauma risk. Susan could not tolerate the thought of tearing again in the same area and the fact that healing could be delayed or complicated. She opted for an elective caesarean section, fully understanding that being in theatre could be a challenge but relieved that she had carefully considered all the options and come to what she felt was the right decision for her particular circumstances. A documented plan was also made that should she labour after 34 weeks gestation, she would still have a caesarean section in order to preserve her perineal and vaginal tissues from trauma. She was shown around the theatre environment to reduce her anxiety as part of the preparation for the birth.

Susan had a healthy boy delivered by elective caesarean section at 39 weeks gestation.

This case illustrates why it is key to understand the actual fears that a particular woman may have. Listening to a history of previous traumatic events, it is easy for clinicians to make incorrect assumptions about the focus of the fear or anxiety. Sometimes the fears can easily be addressed or may even be similar for both a vaginal birth and a caesarean section once a realistic description of what might happen is shared. Women may at first request a caesarean section but subsequently opt for a vaginal birth with the right support over the key issues. In this case, Susan finally opted for a caesarean section because of the scar tissue that remained and the likely risk this posed for problematic healing, which could have resulted in further psychological difficulty, not based on her original reasoning.

Relationship between tocophobia, PTSD and postnatal PTSD

One of the most common causes of tocophobia among multiparous women is a previous traumatic birth. The terms 'traumatic birth' and 'birth trauma' are used loosely by many clinicians and lay people alike. What is often meant by the term 'birth trauma' is that the woman had a 'difficult time' or experienced a 'complication' that left them with some anxiety that may – or may not – be totally rational. In my opinion, these loose terms frequently do not fit the definition for tocophobia, which has an irrational component, or the criteria for diagnosis of postnatal PTSD (PN-PTSD). Clarity is essential.

PN-PTSD can impact significantly on subsequent pregnancies and predispose the woman to future tocophobia. Midwives and obstetricians should be able to identify women who have genuine PN-PTSD and tocophobia. Failure to do so can result in a lack of appropriate referral and failings in appropriate advice, care and management.

PTSD and postnatal PTSD

What is post-traumatic stress disorder?

Post-traumatic stress disorder (PTSD) is classified as an anxiety disorder (APA, 2000, 2013). It is a disorder that can affect people of any age. PTSD may develop after an individual is exposed to a traumatic event such as the threat of death to self or others, serious injury or other catastrophic situations. The individual usually experiences intense fear, horror or powerlessness.

The term PTSD was first used to describe a set of symptoms seen in First World War veterans following horrific experiences. The diagnosis hinges on a set of three key characteristic symptoms: recurring flashbacks, avoidance or numbing of memories and hyper-arousal (NICE, 2005).

- *Re-experiencing symptoms.* Sufferers re-experience aspects of the traumatic event in an involuntary, vivid and distressing way. Flashbacks occur in which the sufferer feels as if experiencing the event all over again. The feelings can cause intense distress and/or physiological symptoms.
- *Avoidance behaviour.* Sufferers avoid people, situations or circumstances that may remind them of the original experience. At the same time, they may ruminate excessively about the event itself and the questions they have surrounding why it happened.
- *Hyper-arousal.* This includes irritability, poor concentration, sleep disorder and hypervigilance for threat. There is also often emotional numbing, a feeling of detachment from others and a lack of interest in other activities.

The diagnosis is further sub-classified according to the length of time the symptoms have been present. Acute PTSD is present if the symptoms have been present less than three months, chronic PTSD if the symptoms have been present three months or more, and delayed-onset PTSD if the symptoms first occur after six months or more. PTSD is distinct from the briefer acute stress disorder, which is of shorter duration. (Acute stress disorder must be resolved within four weeks of the trauma.)

The characteristic symptoms of PTSD must not be present in the individual prior to exposure to the traumatic event for a diagnosis of PTSD to be made.

Causes of PTSD

The majority of people who experience a traumatizing event will not go on to develop PTSD. The average risk of developing PTSD after trauma is approximately 8% for men and 20% for women (25–30% overall) (NICE, 2005). PTSD can occur in people with no pre-existing conditions or risk factors. However, examples of those who are considered to be at risk include military personnel, victims of natural disasters, victims of violent crime, and those who are employed in occupations that expose them to traumatic events such as emergency service workers.

Evidence from the study of twins supports the theory that susceptibility to PTSD is hereditary (True et al., 1993; Skre et al., 2000). Research has also found that PTSD shares many genetic influences common to other psychiatric conditions. Panic and generalized anxiety disorders and PTSD share 60% of the same genetic variance. Alcohol, nicotine and drug dependence share more than 40% genetic similarities (Skelton et al., 2012).

What is postnatal PTSD?

Postnatal PTSD (PN-PTSD) was first described in 1994 when it was recognized as part of the DSM-IV criteria by the American Psychiatric Association (APA, 1994). If a mother responds with intense fear, helplessness or horror to her birthing experience, it is possible she will go on to develop PTSD – specifically classified as PN-PTSD if she experiences the symptom pattern previously described above, persisting for 12 weeks or more.

Many women may suffer similar symptoms (i.e. flashbacks, avoidance behaviour and hyper-arousal) in the early weeks after childbirth. While it is important to recognize these women and be appropriately understanding, the majority of symptoms resolve and they do not go on to have a diagnosis of PN-PTSD. In addition, birth partners, who have or believe they have witnessed a horrific and life-threatening situation during observation of the birth, may also develop PTSD (or arguably PN-PTSD).

What is the cause of PN-PTSD?

Quality research in to this area is lacking. Research previously has focussed on the type of delivery itself. However, the Birth Trauma Association (undated) write extensively about cases which suggest that the degree of distress is often less associated with the event itself but more with the perception of control, the attitudes of people around the birthing couple, relationships with clinicians, information provided and ability to consent. PN-PTSD can occur after any type of delivery, including spontaneous vaginal birth. The Birth Trauma Association report a number of women developing PTSD after home birth. They state that 'a woman's subjective perception of her birth experience is more important than the objective experience itself'. Whether or not a woman experiences her birth as a traumatic event or not is certainly not related to the clinician's perception of whether the birth is or is not traumatic. These findings are consistent with my own practice. All modes of birth and all birth settings give rise to experiences that can lead to PN-PTSD and tocophobia in some women. Midwives and obstetricians need to understand that their own actions and communications, even in the most seemingly 'normal' circumstances, can contribute significantly to these adverse psychological outcomes.

Case 5.2: Aniela

Summary of history

Aniela was 28 years old when she was referred from a community healthcare professional for discussion and debriefing following the birth of her baby four months previously. She had delivered vaginally following an eight-hour labour and 45 minutes of pushing. She had not required pain relief until the midwife used a local anaesthetic to suture a small vaginal tear. She had found the whole experience so traumatizing that she had been unable to discuss it with anyone.

As her story unfolded, it became apparent that she had a longstanding history of vaginismus and only had penetrative sex in the hope of becoming pregnant. This had been extremely painful but at least she had achieved her aim. She described her labour and delivery in graphic terms and tearful detail. This highlighted the fact that, to many, her birth experience might have been deemed 'ideal'. This could not have been further from reality. The fact that she was repeatedly told by healthcare professionals that she had had the 'perfect labour and birth' had added to her anxiety symptoms and flashbacks and concerns about becoming pregnant in the future.

Aniela had a diagnosis of PN-PTSD. Her main flashbacks related to her interactions with several carers during labour and also to times when she was 'left in the room' on her own. She broke down as she expressed her wish that if she became pregnant again, she would choose caesarean section.

Summary of counselling assessment and birth plan
Aniela was seen for counselling over the course of the following year. This included the use of vaginal trainers to help her with the vaginismus. She was able to achieve comfortable and enjoyable penetrative sex and her PN-PTSD was resolved. She was discharged from follow-up.

Two years after the birth of her first child, she was referred back for requesting an elective caesarean section. Once pregnant, she had become fearful of giving birth and some of her anxiety symptoms and flashbacks had returned. After counselling, Aniela, the obstetrician and the lead midwife agreed to careful construction of a birth plan that was communicated to a small team of experienced midwives. These plans addressed the specific issues that were anxiety triggers in her previous experience. Clear boundaries were defined and documented regarding different options should she need assistance or change her mind during labour. Enabling her to have this control avoided unnecessary caesarean section and resulted in a spontaneous vaginal birth with a completely different psychological experience from her first.

What are the consequences of PN-PTSD?

The consequences of PN-PTSD can be far-reaching (Table 5.1). The most immediate issues relate directly to the intensity and length of time the symptoms persist. As can be seen from the description of symptoms, PN-PTSD can affect most aspects of daily living as well as breastfeeding and bonding with the baby. Postnatal isolation is a common consequence. If unrecognized or untreated, some women will go on to develop clinical depression. Some develop issues with alcohol and substance abuse. In the longer term, secondary tocophobia will affect a significant proportion of PN-PTSD sufferers. Although their PTSD symptoms may disappear, once the woman experiences the desire to have another child, the tocophobia will become apparent (Menage, 1993).

The avoidance behaviours characteristic of the symptoms of PTSD mean that women who have PN-PTSD may develop fear of sex in addition to tocophobia.

Table 5.1 Summary of possible consequences of PN-PTSD.

- Depression and ongoing anxiety problems
- Alcohol and substance abuse
- Tocophobia
- Sexual avoidance/dysfunction
- Relationship problems (with partner, family and children)
- Avoidance of medical care (especially smears and intimate examinations)
- Suicide (significant cause of indirect maternal deaths) (CMACE, 2011; Knight et al., 2014)

This can cause relationship issues and distress. They may also avoid screening and treatment for gynaecological issues such as smears and sexually transmitted infections to the detriment of their health. In extreme cases, some women avoid all contact with healthcare professionals for more general issues (Menage, 1993).

Practice point

Midwives and obstetricians need to have a working knowledge of tocophobia and PN-PTSD to give women with these conditions the best care in pregnancy and childbirth. Listening to and then interpreting the woman's story are the key skills required.

Impact of tocophobia and PN-PTSD on normal birth

If PN-PTSD and/or tocophobia are poorly managed or unrecognized in pregnancy care, it will impact on labour and birth in a subsequent pregnancy. Satisfaction, anxiety and mode of birth will be affected. If poorly managed, some women may not present until labour when it becomes very challenging to support their anxiety issues effectively. Others may request elective caesarean section and be offered it without thought to the real underlying issues, which could possibly have been addressed. The outcome is that some women have unnecessary caesarean sections. Obstetricians and midwives influence some women by suggesting that they have a caesarean to 'relieve' their anxiety and fear when the woman had not even considered this might be necessary. All these factors increase the elective caesarean section rate and decrease the vaginal birth rate. (These rates are very difficult to quantify with accuracy, as the topic lacks good quality research.)

   If tocophobia and PN-PTSD are recognized and well managed, some women will opt for vaginal birth, some will opt for caesarean section and others will change their mind about the right mode of delivery for them later in their pregnancies. The majority of women who change their mind are women who initially requested caesarean section but who then opt for vaginal birth. In an audit in my own birth trauma clinic of women requesting elective caesarean section because of PN-PTSD, following counselling 63% chose to plan for a vaginal birth. Of these, 43% achieved a vaginal birth and 18% had a caesarean section for obstetric indications.

In summary, if women who have PN-PTSD or tocophobia are well managed by midwives and obstetricians working in genuine collaboration, this will improve the vaginal birth rate in this group. In turn, this will improve long-term obstetric outcomes. Those women who continue to opt for caesarean section feel empowered and in control. I would also argue that all have better outcomes in terms of PN-PTSD and depression but there is limited, if any, good evidence to support or challenge this view.

Tocophobia in the context of NICE guidance and caesarean section

The latest NICE guidance (NICE, 2011b) regarding caesarean section acknowledges that psychological fear of childbirth is an issue for some women. Although the guidance recommends caesarean section be on offer, there is considerable ambiguity in its statements. This ambiguity has created an unintended consequence and a new challenge for clinicians: the perception that caesarean on demand is endorsed by NICE and that is also regularly confused with tocophobia or psychological issues. The consequence is rising unnecessary caesarean section rates.

In the context of this chapter, the challenge facing clinicians is to consider which women really do have tocophobia (an abnormal fear) in the true sense of the definition and which have a 'normal fear' of childbirth. Where resources are scarce, clearly the tocophobic group need more help and input than those with a more 'normal fear', who can be helped by antenatal education, friends and family, and are unlikely to suffer long-term consequences of their fears. Difficult prioritization decisions may have to be made. Within the tocophobic group, a caesarean section is right for some and a vaginal birth for others. A dangerous misinterpretation of the NICE guidance would be to recommend that all women with tocophobia should be offered a caesarean section. These women are different from the women who simply request a caesarean section for convenience. Careful assessment on an individual basis with the involvement of obstetricians and midwives experienced in psychological issues should ensure that the right women have the right birth plan for the right reasons. Clear documentation is essential.

Caesarean section as a matter of convenience is not the key issue here. The real issue is about ensuring that women with a genuine fear of childbirth are not given a caesarean section for the wrong reason or forced down a pathway of normal birth with possible adverse long-term psychological consequences that could have been avoided.

> **Practice point**
>
> Units where midwives and obstetricians can together provide a genuinely collaborative service for women with tocophobia and PN-PTSD will improve the normal birth rate and reduce unnecessary caesarean sections in this group.

Antenatal assessment of women with tocophobia/PN-PTSD

There is no 'right way' or protocol for the antenatal assessment of women with tocophobia/PN-PTSD; there is no 'one approach fits all'. Two key words that would apply to all settings would be 'listen' and 'interpret'. Listening skills among healthcare professionals are improving but it is more challenging to acquire skills of interpretation.

When caring for women with known tocophobia or a referral containing an assumed tocophobia, there are some common steps along the pregnancy pathway that should form part of a good assessment; these are outlined in Box 5.2.

> **Box 5.2: Assessment of women with tocophobia or suspected tocophobia**
>
> 1   Clarify and understand what the particular fears of the woman are. Determine if anything specific is being requested. During the first meeting, it is essential to listen to the woman's story, allowing her time to articulate all the important issues. Referral letters can make inappropriate or incorrect assumptions that colour the clinician's view from the outset before even speaking to the woman concerned. A correct description of the issues may be presented in a referral but followed by an incorrect set of requests. These can represent the requests of the referrer and not the woman.
> 2   Consider whether any requests are rational or irrational. Determine whether the requests can/should be accommodated. Sometimes a woman will make a request based on an incorrect assumption. Understanding her rationale allows appropriate discussion and sometimes results in a withdrawal of the request or change of mind. It is important to distinguish the difference between 'normal' and 'abnormal' fear. This should be achieved early on in order to allocate resources and time to those who most need it.
> 3   Assess the need for further expert help and referral. This may be to an obstetrician with a specialized interest and/or experienced midwife in the field. Input from a psychosexual counsellor or perinatal psychiatrist may be required in specific cases for appropriate therapy (psychological or medical).

4   To deliver optimum care to this group of women, **real** collaboration between midwives and obstetricians together with an understanding of tocophobia is essential: these women cannot successfully be looked after by midwives or obstetricians alone. They need each other and the woman needs both. This is because one cannot foresee how events will unfold. Ideally, there should be a team of interested and knowledgeable midwives and obstetricians who regularly care for such women and referral pathways should be clear. Other colleagues also need to understand the key issues and support any plans that are made.

5   Clinicians must understand that this will be a *process* and that decisions regarding care are unlikely to be satisfactorily reached in one consultation or interaction. A key issue for most women with tocophobia is the need to be in control. Clinicians need to facilitate this woman-led control wherever possible. Control will be maximized by allowing women time to consider what has been discussed away from the clinical setting and then further opportunities for discussion. For most women, it is important that they have the opportunity to meet a member from each of the midwifery and obstetric teams.

6   The most important aspect of planning for most women with tocophobia is a negotiated and clear birth and postnatal plan that addresses their specific fears. Realistic expectations must also be set, and the making of promises that cannot be followed through avoided. The woman must have confidence that plans will be followed. Units where midwives and doctors work independently of each other are likely to cause more issues for women with tocophobia. Both must sometimes work outside of their 'comfort zone' and be flexible according to the woman's needs. Units where there is a team of clinicians who are experienced and sympathetic to dealing with tocophobia can provide excellent individualized care in a planned way.

7   Postnatal follow-up and counselling should be offered where appropriate or if there are ongoing issues. There is no evidence that one-off debriefing for PN-PTSD is beneficial (NICE, 2005).

Caesarean section request: case-based summary examples

The following examples describe three different women with tocophobia, each of whom requested an elective caesarean section.

•   Hannah's underlying fear was to do with feeling exposed. This had been triggered by the way she felt that the obstetrician had exposed her during her first birth, which resulted in an instrumental delivery in a labour ward. Once she had a full understanding of the obstetric theatre and the people who worked there, she chose to plan for a vaginal birth whereby she would be cared for by one midwife. If there were to be any complications, she was familiar with the theatre setting and procedure and had visited it twice.

- Shelley's underlying fear was of a potential lack of examination in labour and that the obstetricians might *not* be involved in care and progress. This had resulted from a previous bad experience where progress in labour had been delayed and had not been appropriately identified, resulting in caesarean section. The woman was reassured of collaboration, seen jointly by a lead midwife and obstetrician, and a careful birth plan created together. This included regular four-hourly examinations in active labour and commitment to discussions within the team about progress. Shelley achieved a vaginal birth.

- Fatima's underlying fear was in fact unrelated to her previous birth experience but directly related to her perceived previous lack of care on postnatal wards. Once introduced to the postnatal team, with a commitment from them to provide more input postnatally, she was confident enough to opt for a vaginal birth rather than pursue her request for caesarean section.

The above scenarios sound quick and simple when put in writing. The reality is that it takes considerable time and skill to draw out the real issues and fears and to put plans in place. Some women's anxiety is so great that they cannot deviate from their initial request for caesarean section even after multiple clinic sessions. Some women, though traumatized, are not able to articulate their specific underlying fears until they are drawn out and interpreted by an experienced therapist. It is only then that they can make some logical decisions regarding what may help and what mode of birth or plan of care is 'right' for them.

What can clinicians do to improve birth experiences and reduce the incidence of tocophobia/PN-PTSD?

To address this question, consideration needs to be given to all aspects of the pregnancy care pathway. Midwives, doctors and other healthcare professionals can make a difference at every stage. The actions taken in one pregnancy will affect the choices that women make in subsequent pregnancies.

There are four key factors that influence a woman's childbirth experience:

1   Personal expectations (including antenatal classes and realistic information)
2   The amount of support during labour and birth
3   The quality of the relationship between the woman and her caregivers
4   The woman's involvement in decision-making (perceived and actual).

All women come to labour and birth with some ability to handle discomfort, decrease stress and cope based on their previous life experiences. These life experiences cannot be altered but health professionals can influence the current key factors and enable women to learn new strategies to improve their childbirth experience.

Practice point

Some women will experience tocophobia or PN-PTSD regardless of skill, collaboration, expertise and optimization of care. However, some women will be spared this trauma or have a better subsequent birth experience through improved knowledge, experience and training of clinicians.

Conclusion

It is clear that, for some women, fear of childbirth has an enormous impact on their lives. This fear is most pronounced perhaps among those women who are never seen in maternity care because they have been unable to overcome their fear enough to become pregnant. For others, health professionals contribute to the cause of their fear in different ways.

Communication is a word that all healthcare professionals are familiar with and yet women continue to remind us in feedback surveys that we frequently fall short. Obstetricians and midwives must seek to understand those whom we care for at this crucial and emotional time of their lives. We must individualize care and help women to feel confident, comfortable and supported through childbirth experiences. This would prevent some women from experiencing PN-PTSD or tocophobia. It needs to be recognized that individuals with such diagnoses will require more from us and our service during subsequent pregnancies. Increased attention to the training and education of our clinical teams with regard to understanding tocophobia would benefit all the women we serve.

Both tocophobia and PN-PTSD have an impact on mode of birth. Incorrect assumptions (by both women and clinicians) that a caesarean section will be the best solution are regularly seen in practice. Although a caesarean section may be the most appropriate choice for some, it is not the case for all. Often the decision for caesarean section is made without real thought given to understanding the underlying issues, which might have been resolved by adopting alternative plans. In some cases, performing a caesarean section still expose the woman to her real fears and issues and the psychological symptoms can worsen. (Furthermore, she will have had a caesarean section with all the future implications that implies.) Equally disturbing are cases where women are 'encouraged' to choose a vaginal birth option against their wishes, with attendant worsening anxiety and phobic symptoms.

Obstetricians and midwives must work closely together to serve this group of women in the best way they can. Women with tocophobia need specialized input and collaborative care plans that are clearly understood and supported by the wider team. Working independently as obstetricians or as midwives will not serve this group optimally; collaborative working is required if the desire is to improve outcome.

High-quality research on the impact of tocophobia on normal birth is very difficult to conduct. With regard to 'outcomes', we ought not to be motivated by overall 'numbers' but the experience of individuals and their psychological well-being going forward. If research could demonstrate a reduction in the number of caesarean sections, this would be an excellent but secondary outcome. Collectively, our passion should be to help people achieve positive experiences of childbirth irrespective of mode of birth or any complications that may arise.

Further reading

Beck, C. (2004) Birth trauma is in the eye of the beholder, *Nurse Research*, 53 (1): 28–35. An interesting phenomenological study that examines the subjective nature of what clinicians and women consider 'good' or 'traumatic' births.

Robinson, J. (2007) Post traumatic stress disorder, *AIMS Journal*, 19 (1). An excellent article which explores the history, the diagnosis and treatment of PTSD. Includes some of the challenges of these aspects of PTSD.

References

American Psychiatric Association (APA) (1994) *Diagnostic and Statistical Manual of Mental Disorders: DSM-IV.* Washington, DC: American Psychiatric Association.

American Psychiatric Association (APA) (2000) *Diagnostic and Statistical Manual of Mental Disorders, Fourth Edition, Text Revision (DSM-IV-TR).* Washington, DC: American Psychiatric Association.

American Psychiatric Association (APA) (2013) *Diagnostic and Statistical Manual of Mental Disorders, Fifth Edition (DSM-V).* Washington, DC: American Psychiatric Association.

Birth Trauma Association (undated) *Post Natal Post Traumatic Stress Disorder.* Ipswich: BTA [http://www.birthtraumaassociation.org.uk/publications/Post_Natal_PTSD.pdf].

Centre for Maternal and Child Enquiries (CMACE) (2011) Saving mothers' lives – Reviewing maternal deaths to make motherhood safer: 2006–2008. The Eighth Report of the confidential enquiries into maternal deaths in the United Kingdom, *BJOG: An International Journal of Obstetrics and Gynaecology*, 118 (suppl.1): 1–203.

Collins Dictionary (2016) www.collinsdictionary.com/dictionary/english/tocophobia [accessed 10/ March 2016].

Curtis, G.C., Magee, W.J., Eaton, W.W., Wittchen, H.U. and Kessier, R.C. (1998) Specific fears and phobias: epidemiology and classification, *British Journal of Psychiatry*, 173: 212–17.

Encyclo (2016) http://www.encyclo.co.uk/meaning-of-Tocophobia [accessed 10 March 2016].

Fyer, A.J., Mannuzza, S., Gallops M.S., Martin, L.Y., Aaronson, C., Gorman, J.M. et al. (1990) Familial transmission of simple phobias and fears: a preliminary report, *Archives of General Psychiatry*, 47 (3): 252–6.

Geissbuehel, V. and Eberhand, J. (2002) Fear of childbirth during pregnancy: a study of more than 8000 pregnant women, *Journal of Psychosomatic Obstetrics and Gynecology*, 23: 229–35.

Hofberg, K. and Brockington, I. (2000) Tocophobia: an unreasoning dread of childbirth. A series of 26 cases, *British Journal of Psychiatry*, 176: 83–5.

Hofberg, K. and Ward, M. (2003) Fear of childbirth, *Postgraduate Medical Journal*, 79: 505–10.

Kendler, K.S., Karkowski, L.M. and Prescott, C.A. (1999) Fears and phobias: reliability and heritability, *Psychological Medicine*, 29 (3): 539–53.

Knight, M., Kenyon, S., Brocklehurst, P., Neilson, J., Shakespeare, J. and Kurinczuk, J.J. (eds) (2014) *Saving Lives, Improving Mothers' Care: Lessons learned to inform future maternity care from the UK and Ireland Confidential Enquiries into Maternal Deaths and Morbidity 2009–12*. Oxford: National Perinatal Epidemiology Unit, University of Oxford [http://www.npeu.ox.ac.uk/downloads/files/mbrrace-uk/reports/Saving%20Lives%20Improving%20Mothers%20Care%20report%202014%20Full.pdf].

McCabe, R.E., Ashbaugh, A.R. and Antony, M.M. (2010) Specific and social phobias, in M.M. Antony and D.H. Barlow (eds) *Handbook of Assessment and Treatment Planning for Psychological Disorders* (2nd edn). New York: Guilford Press.

Menage, J. (1993) Post-traumatic stress disorder in women who have undergone obstetric and/or gynaecological procedures, *Journal of Reproductive and Infant Psychology*, 11: 221–8.

National Institute for Health and Care Excellence (NICE) (2005) *Post-traumatic Stress Disorder: Management*, Clinical Guideline CG26. Manchester: NICE [https://www.nice.org.uk/guidance/cg26].

National Institute for Health and Care Excellence (NICE) (2009) *Depression in Adults: Recognition and management*, Clinical Guideline CG90. Manchester: NICE [https://www.nice.org.uk/guidance/cg90].

National Institute for Health and Care Excellence (NICE) (2011a) *Generalised Anxiety Disorder and Panic Disorder in Adults: Management*, Clinical Guideline CG113. Manchester: NICE [https://www.nice.org.uk/guidance/cg113].

National Institute for Health and Care Excellence (NICE) (2011b) *Caesarean Section*, Clinical Guideline CG132. Manchester: NICE [https://www.nice.org.uk/guidance/cg132].

Skelton, K., Ressler, K.J., Norrholm, S.D., Jovanovic, T. and Bradley-Davino, B. (2012) PTSD and gene variants: new pathways and new thinking, *Neuropharmacology*, 62 (2): 628–37.

Skre, I., Onstad, S., Torgersen, S., Phiulos, D.R., Lygren, S. and Kringlen, E. (2000) The heritability of common phobic fear: a twin study of a clinical sample, *Journal of Anxiety Disorders*, 14 (6): 549–62.

True, W.R., Rice, J. and Eisen, S.A. (1993) A twin study of genetic and environmental contributions to liability for posttraumatic stress symptoms, *Archives of General Psychiatry*, 50 (4): 257–64.

Waldenström, U., Hildingsson, I.M. and Ryding, E.L. (2006) Antenatal fear of childbirth and its association with subsequent caesarean section and experience of childbirth, *BJOG: An International Journal of Obstetrics and Gynaecology*, 113 (6): 638–46.

Wijma, K. (2003) Why focus on 'fear of childbirth'?, *Journal of Psychosomatic Obstetrics and Gynecology*, 24 (3): 141–3.

6

Latent phase of labour
What makes latent phase complicated?
Helen Spiby

Introduction

Latent phase labour was traditionally framed as a natural precursor to the established component of first stage labour. Historically, it received scant attention in midwifery texts and for most women it proceeded away from professional observation and input, at home, often supported by female relatives and companions.

This chapter, part of a book about complicated or challenging childbirth, will explore some aspects of the phenomenon of latent phase labour. It will consider *complicated* latent phase labour in a range of ways. First, an attempt is made to define 'latent phase', followed by an overview of midwifery care organization and content in the latent phase. Next, I explore why some healthcare professionals and women consider latent phase labour to be *complicated* and, finally, provide suggestions for the next phase of early labour research.

Defining latent phase labour

It is often stated that to understand a phenomenon, it is first necessary to define it. Where labour is concerned, definitions of 'complicated' often focus on the measurable and in terms of labour, this equates to length. However, to adopt this approach immediately causes difficulty by reducing the latent phase to one characteristic, when contemporary childbearing is most optimally located within a social context and where process does not dominate (Walsh, 2006). If, however, duration of the latent phase is seen as a potential type of complicated labour, further challenges emerge. It is widely acknowledged that the exact point of onset of labour can never be known, as it is not an event but a process, initiated by a complex range of factors, including some that may not yet be fully understood. Recent research has systematically reviewed the range of definitions of labour onset and identified a plethora of definitions of the onset of labour overall – including that for first stage onset and latent phase onset – all based on scant evidence (Hanley et al., 2015). The latent phase is therefore immediately complicated by lack of clarity of definition. This appears mainly as an issue for nulliparous women due to newness of experience and also for those supporting and caring for them.

Without clarity of definition of onset, it is difficult to set criteria for either prolonged or the seldom considered, rapid latent phase. Research related to a prolonged latent phase must therefore be interpreted in the context of uncertainty and different definitions. While Dixon and colleagues (2013) demonstrated that women do not frame labour by stages, clarity around onset of latent phase and established first stage of labour must be achieved by those providing clinical care to avoid inappropriate intervention or diagnosis of poor progress.

Guidelines recently published by the American College of Obstetricians and Gynaecologists (ACOG, 2014) based on a re-evaluation of data related to labour progress, have been accepted in North America, relatively unopposed. The significance of these guidelines for latent labour is in the redefining of established labour onset at 6 cm cervical dilatation, rather than the previously accepted definition of 3–4 cm cervical dilatation.

Providing midwifery care in the latent phase

Until relatively recently, little research focused on how care should be provided to women in latent phase labour. Early in the current millennium, studies began to emerge from England, Scotland, Canada, Sweden and Germany that focused on latent rather than subsequent labour stages. They appear to have been prompted by a number of concerns, including rising rates of intervention, instrumental and operative births. Some retrospective studies in a range of settings indicated that early admission to central labour suites appeared to be associated with increased rates of intervention during labour (Hemminki and Simukka, 1986; Holmes et al., 2001) and associated increased morbidity. In addition, there was an increasing understanding of how women experience labour onset (Gross et al., 2003), and the gap between women's experiences and how labour onset has traditionally been framed by maternity professionals (Gross et al., 2009). In Canada, some interventions tested in pilot studies appeared promising. These included a small trial that evaluated care provided away from a main labour suite (McNiven et al., 1998), and Janssen and colleagues' (2003) pilot trial of home visiting in early labour.

In the UK, concerns about rising rates of intervention during labour, meeting women's needs for support and assessment, and significant numbers of category X admissions (women admitted, assessed and found not to be in labour and discharged home or to await established labour on the antenatal ward) triggered studies in England and Wales (Spiby et al., 2007, 2008). It was acknowledged that women in early or latent phase of labour required support and assessment but providing such care on a main labour ward was considered to compromise the care available to women in established labour. In Scotland, a cluster trial explored use of an algorithm to support diagnosis of labour as a support-tool for midwives' decision-making of labour onset (Cheyne et al., 2008). The implications for the latent phase arising from some of these studies will be explored below. The extent of this activity within a few years and initiated by independent research groups must surely reflect a phenomenon that is less than straightforward and indeed quite complex.

The process and organization of care

A range of approaches exists to provide care for women in latent phase labour. Traditionally, as a first step in the care process, the majority of women planning birth in a maternity unit have been expected to telephone the unit where they were planning to give birth and subsequently to travel to the unit for face-to-face assessment. The telephone conversation is generally held to perform several functions. From the perspectives of the organization, there is foreknowledge of a woman's admission, enabling workload allocation and unit capacity to be considered, the opportunity to appraise labour onset, progress, emotional wellbeing and to obtain medical records, prepare a room and allocate a caregiver. From the woman's perspectives, the conversation may include seeking or providing information about labour onset and progress, obtaining reassurance of normality and information about coping, and when to travel to the maternity unit. Unfortunately in this assessment process, most women have had to interact with midwives whom they have not previously met and with whom there is no established relationship. For the midwives involved, there is often access to only minimal information about the woman's particular circumstances. The exceptions to this include models of care where high levels of continuity are provided, such as caseload and some team midwifery schemes. In addition, midwives will be taking telephone calls in busy and often relatively public areas, generally interspersed with other clinical, educational and administrative responsibilities.

As part of a suite of early labour studies, a survey of Heads of Midwifery in England, carried out in 2004/5, identified a range of approaches to early labour service provision there (Spiby et al., 2007). Almost half of the units (49%) reported changes to their early labour service provision over the previous 5 years, and a quarter reported that they were planning further changes. These approaches, which in many cases removed the activity of early labour assessment from the main labour ward, were initiated by a number of factors, including responding to service user feedback and new clinical policies, but most often changes were initiated due to concerns about category X admissions. The systems of early labour care identified in the survey included: telephone and face-to-face triage approaches, sometimes conducted in newly opened triage areas, the opening of maternity assessment units and revised documentation to support assessment. The amount of service change identified in the survey was extensive but perhaps surprisingly, many units found it difficult to provide exact figures for category X admissions, a key trigger for change. In addition, while the new approaches were reported as generally positive from the services' perspective, relatively little monitoring of early labour services and activity was reported (Spiby et al., 2013). This dearth of evaluation and data demonstrates the uncertainty inherent in current latent phase labour care.

Providing care by telephone

A few years before the start of our early labour research, the NHS in England introduced a telephone service, NHS Direct, initially as a pilot in 1998 and more widely in 2000 (Commission for Health Improvement, 2004). This service, introduced to reduce the demands made on primary care, was staffed by qualified nurses who provided advice based on algorithmically driven conversations with patients. In our research, we enquired whether Heads of Midwifery services thought there was a potential role for NHS Direct in early labour services; slightly fewer than 10% agreed. Only four services had explored this and none had proceeded to implement it. Concerns around this related most frequently to the need for advice to be provided by a midwife; negative implications for communications and continuity for women; and a view that women's needs would best be met by healthcare professionals aware of each Trust's own protocols and the needs of women in their catchment area. Other midwives saw a threat to the midwifery role and to the quality of advice provided (Spiby et al., 2007).

The All Wales Pathway for Normal Labour and Birth, based on an integrated care pathway, comprised three components to the care plan, the first of which focused on the telephone conversations made by women to their maternity unit in early labour (Ferguson, 2004). The aim of the Pathway was that, following assessment of labour, the midwife would offer a woman evidence-based advice on remaining at home or being admitted to the maternity unit. Forty-six women provided detailed information about their experiences of those calls in computer-assisted telephone interviews. Women's experiences of those telephone conversations revealed some dissatisfaction and unmet needs (Green et al., 2012). Some women were dissatisfied about several aspects. Specifically, women were more likely to be dissatisfied if the advice they received was unclear, if their needs were not met during the telephone call, if anxieties remained unaddressed at the end of the call and if the midwife's manner was not deemed to be positive. The shortness of calls also featured as a source of dissatisfaction; in particular, women whose calls lasted less than 5 minutes were more likely to be dissatisfied. Women appreciated clear advice about the next steps, when to telephone again or when to travel to the maternity unit. They also valued midwives who provided reassurance and information, were friendly and encouraging and sounded confident. However, some women felt uncomfortable following calls and that their concerns had been trivialized. Feeling they were welcome to go into the maternity unit was an important factor in women's satisfaction, even if they did not feel the need to travel at that time. The relationship between women and their midwives in the latent phase may become problematic due to poor communication and misunderstanding of advice and the rationale behind it.

Recent additions to the range of approaches for early labour telephone conversations in England include calls being taken by community midwives, working from a base away from the main labour suite where their advice is provided unaffected by the workload of the maternity unit. Local evaluation reflected women's satisfaction with this system (Weavers and Nash, 2012). In a different Trust, an initiative where midwives take early labour calls from a base in an NHS ambulance station is being evaluated (Nott and Pragnell, 2015).

Currently, there is considerable pressure on UK maternity services: midwifery shortages, increasing case complexity and an increasing birth rate. There are occasions when women are unable to birth in their planned unit and may only be informed of this at the point of telephone contact in labour. It is important that the needs of these women are considered and that a high-quality dialogue is conducted in what, for many women and their companions, will be an anxiety provoking situation. Research conducted in Sweden among women who were required at labour onset to travel to a unit other than that planned due to lack of space, holds salutary information for midwives providing care in such situations. Women who had to transfer resorted to more pharmacological pain relief and were more likely to feel that referral to a different unit to that planned had affected their emotional state (Wiklund et al., 2002).

For every telephone call, there are at least two perspectives related to early labour. Following identification of features of women's experience of telephone conversations, it seemed appropriate to explore midwives' concerns and experiences about early labour calls too. In a small qualitative study, midwives' beliefs and concerns about early labour telephone conversations were explored (Spiby et al., 2014). This research reflected some of the findings of earlier research, namely that a key role for delivery suite midwives is that of gatekeepers to women's access to the clinical area (Cheyne et al., 2006). This aspect of their responsibilities exists concurrently with those of providing support to individual women and the tensions created can contribute to midwives' stress. Midwives identified information deficits for women, especially around latent phase labour due to a perceived reduction in the availability of antenatal education. Their perspective was to encourage women to remain at home, believing that this was in the women's best interests but acknowledged the lack of variation in advice given to women telephoning the maternity unit. Further work is needed that explores perspectives of telephone conversations from both parties to the same call.

One of the fundamental issues on which midwives' responses differ is whether labour onset can be confirmed by telephone conversations alone. Midwives' views vary: some midwives feel that this cannot be achieved (Spiby et al., 2007) whereas others believe that telephone conversations provide a relatively complete means of assessment (Spiby et al., 2014).

Triage

The early use of triage systems was in battlefield medicine, with a focus on prioritizing treatment of casualties who could return to active service. Subsequently transferred into hospital medicine in the 1950s to manage pressures on North American emergency rooms, reports appeared from the maternity context in the 1990s, also in North American settings. In the survey of early labour services carried out in England in 2005, 13% of units, excluding birth centres, reported the existence of triage units. Where triage areas had been introduced, positive impacts on managing workload were seen quite quickly in some settings. However, not all triage schemes had been successful and some had been discontinued due to difficulties of location and relationships between staff in the triage area and the main delivery suite (Spiby et al., 2007).

Midwifery home visits

Home visiting in early labour had traditionally been offered in the Domino (domiciliary in-and-out) model of care and in community-based team or caseload midwifery systems (Flint, 1993, 1996). In early research, women booked at a GP unit where home assessment was one component of the care package, used less pharmacological pain relief, had fewer epidurals, less electronic monitoring and interventions during labour than women who gave birth at a consultant unit (Klein et al., 1983). By the mid-2000s, home assessment on a 24-hour a day basis was available in only seven services for all women (Spiby et al., 2007).

A randomized controlled trial of home visiting for women in early labour who were expecting their first baby was carried out in England between 2004 and 2006. Community midwife visits for early labour were available between 08.00 and 21.00 hours. The offer of a community midwifery home visit did not, however, reduce instrumental and operative births for women randomly allocated to receive one (Spiby et al., 2008). This may have been due to the lack of effect on delaying hospital admission and perhaps an interpretation of the intervention as more focused on assessment than support. Although no improvements in clinical outcomes were detected, there was no increase in the risk of complications for women and their babies, including babies born before their mother's arrival at the maternity unit.

Women's experiences of the home visit were obtained in a postal questionnaire completed a few weeks after the birth of their babies. Women reported that midwives were with them in their own home most commonly for between 30 minutes and one hour (52%); 32% reported a visit of less than 30 minutes and 14% of the respondents reported visits lasting more than an hour. The advice received from the midwife who visited included: comfortable positions for labour, advice on nutrition and keeping hydrated; coping strategies and when to travel to hospital. Three-quarters of women reported that all of the advice received was helpful and a further 23% that some of it was helpful; only 2% of respondents failed to find the midwife's advice helpful. Women provided further information about their experiences of home visits in response to three open questions:

1. *What did you like about having a home visit?*
Among the positive features, women ascribed a home visit as enabling them to feel better informed about labour and its progress and to remain in their own home for longer, feeling more confident about coping, and knowing what to expect and when to go into the hospital. Women who were visited by a midwife they had met previously commented as follows:

> As I had already been sent home from the hospital, it was reassuring to have a midwife say that I was ready to go back again and to tell me how I was progressing. [#92]

> Seeing a friendly face. Reassurance that I was doing okay. Time to ask questions before going to hospital. Would have gone earlier if she had not visited, as was lacking in my ability to cope with pain and whole labour. [#2596]

2. *What else would you have liked from a home visit?*
At the time of this research, midwives were trying to reduce the number of vaginal examinations a woman might experience during labour. One of the issues that emerged, reflected in the comments of several women, was that they had expected the midwife to perform a vaginal examination and were surprised when they did not:

> Was told she would not examine me as 'just niggling' but felt I would have preferred confirmation I was x centimetres, even if only 1 or 2. [#1182]

> In retrospect, a vaginal examination would have been good because I was 9 cm dilated when I got to hospital. [#4315]

3. *What did you not like about having a home visit?*
The most common response was 'nothing'. Some of the issues reflect comments above:

> The midwife was rather unwilling to check how dilated I was and kept using excuses why not to check, for example, infection, painful. But she agreed to check me and I felt encouraged once checked, as I was further on than thought. [#3258]

> Just would have preferred her to come slightly quicker but appreciate she was in the middle of a clinic when I first rang. [#1546]

> Some pain relief . . . so I could have stayed home longer. [#2009]

One approach to care will not meet the needs of all women:

> Although the midwife was friendly, we felt that she did not really make any difference to us and that the visit did not really help. [#4521]

Since the millennium, latent phase labour has been receiving much more attention in the form of service change and research in a number of countries. The fact that so much research has focused on this area suggests that the latent phase is complex or, at least, not straightforward, in ways that were not previously recognized. Undoubtedly, concerns about increasing rates of labour interventions and links with rising caesarean section rates have contributed to this. The challenge of achieving individualized care that meets women's needs in high-pressure environments must also be a factor. However, other considerations merit acknowledgement. Contributing to an international round table discussion, Nolan (2009) suggests that women's needs in the latent phase reflect the fact that other key events of pregnancy have passed into medical control, thus eroding women's confidence, resulting in the view that labour has only started when a professional confirms it has. In addition, midwives believe that too little information is available to women and their families regarding the events and course of the latent phase and ascribe this to a perceived reduction in NHS antenatal education (Spiby et al., 2014). Emerging evidence from antenatal education research reflects inadequate preparation for the early stages of labour for women and their male partners, perceptions that have been echoed in focus groups by midwives who regularly provide intrapartum care (Spiby et al., 2015).

The language used to greet women in the latent phase or to describe their situation also requires consideration. In the 1980s, Hunt and Symonds' ethnographic study of a labour ward reflected certain typologies used to categorize women and their labours Those in early labour were referred to as 'nigglers', women who did not appear to merit midwifery attention until further into established labour (Hunt and Symonds, 1995). As illustrated in the women's quotes above, this term persists. However, subtle changes in terminology are appearing. Previously, the term early labour was commonly used, whereas contemporary discussion and guidance favour use of the term 'latent'. It is not yet clear whether women derive different understandings from those terms. What would appear important is that the language used should reflect the significance of the event for women and not trivialize their concerns or situation. More recently in Sweden, Carlsson and colleagues (2009) suggested that women may wish to yield responsibility for their wellbeing to a professional during latent labour and that they are frustrated by unclear information about likely timescales. Eri and colleagues (2010) reported women need to believe there are credible grounds for their admission on the labour ward, perhaps reflecting the sociological theory of 'candidacy' for healthcare (Dixon-Woods et al., 2006). The above seem to reflect both the difficulty of identifying appropriate terminology and the lack of importance accorded to this phase of labour; these factors complicate latent phase communication.

Research questions: avoiding a complicated latent phase

Much recent research has focused on the needs and experiences of women expecting their first babies. This emphasis has generally been supported by the fact that first labours are usually longer and obviously a new experience for the woman. A significant proportion of first labours are induced; women whose first labour is induced may remain unclear about what to experience in the latent phase in a subsequent labour. It is therefore important that needs related to latent labour for women expecting second and subsequent births are not overlooked.

Perceptions of normality may be changing with respect to spontaneous rupture of membranes prior to established labour. While previously considered within the range of ways in which a labour may start, concerns about the potential for infection have resulted in more closely managed approaches and ever-tightening timeframes within which women's labours *should* become established. Different approaches to managing this situation have been explored: immediate induction versus a period of expectant management either at home or in the maternity unit (Martin and Jomeen, 2004), and a variety of different pharmacological agents (Hannah et al., 1996). However, it is 20 years since Hannah and colleagues reported their international randomized controlled trial and despite the quality of that trial, it may be timely to re-evaluate approaches to care. In addition, new products are available that differentiate between amniotic fluid and urinary leakage and a more robust evidence base is required prior to their more widespread introduction; that evidence should include exploration of women's views.

It remains a widely held belief that women should be supported to remain outside hospital in the latent stage of labour and that admission is best when labour has become truly established. While randomized controlled trials conducted to date have yet to see clear differences in delaying hospital admission, new approaches that provide women with reassurance, information and clinical assessment should be evaluated. The contribution of newer forms of communication such as video-calling technology merit investigation.

Ways to support women to cope in the latent phase require further consideration. Admission to the maternity unit and moving between early stage and birth rooms was identified as a disruption to women's use of taught coping strategies (Spiby et al., 2003). One finding from a trial of self-hypnosis for intrapartum pain identified some unexpected consequences for women who had prepared for labour using that method (Finlayson et al., 2015). Women perceived that midwives were less likely to believe that they were in labour due to the state of calmness achieved. While positive for women's coping, this may require education for midwives and healthcare providers to ensure that appraisal of labour onset and progress is not compromised.

Several studies have reported a fairly ubiquitous approach to the advice provided to women who telephone maternity units in latent phase labour. Advice such as 'having a bath' and 'taking two paracetamol', and encouraging remaining at home until labour is established have been reported in studies conducted in a number of settings. Women do not always find this advice helpful (Spiby et al., 2008) and midwives also acknowledge that it may not demonstrate an individualized approach to care (Spiby et al., 2014).

Questions remain about who is the most appropriate person to support women in the latent phase and how those individuals should best be prepared for their role. It remains likely that women will continue to access both family and friends and maternity services for that. Existing evidence suggests that the family and friends who support women in latent phase labour are uncomfortable and lack confidence in that role (Barnett et al., 2008), and that they may require more specific information and preparation. If the recommendations of the American College of Obstetrics and Gynaecology are adopted widely, there may be implications for women and their families in this regard, if a longer period at home ensues. While a randomized controlled trial testing the revised guidelines is in progress in Norway, questions arise as to the implications for women, their families and their caregivers. First, is there an implication that women should remain outside the main labour ward until 6 cm dilatation, and second, how can women, their families and healthcare professionals be assisted to achieve this in a way that meets everyone's needs? It is difficult to see how these different needs can be met without the provision of additional resources to latent phase labour – whether those are human, financial, educational or communication support, or a combination thereof. It is also clear from existing evidence that one approach will not meet all women's needs, but that these resources must be readily accessible to women in the latent phase and thus need to be based or useable in a community rather than institutional location. This is increasingly relevant at a time when, in some areas, women whose labours are induced may be offered the option of returning home, following administration of pharmacological agents, to await established labour. Whether spontaneous in onset or induced, latent phase labour has the potential to be of several hours' duration and to be a source of considerable discomfort, pain and anxiety. New research is needed that focuses on preparing women for those experiences and in developing a toolkit of techniques that can be used during latent phase labour whether women are in their own homes or a maternity unit. Current intrapartum guidelines reflect the range of places where women may give birth (NICE, 2014). Any new approaches developed for early labour need also to have utility for the range of settings where women may subsequently experience established labour and birth.

There is growing evidence of the contribution of peer supporters across a number of fields of healthcare. In maternity, the contribution is especially established for breastfeeding and more broadly in the approaches that support women with particular needs in the development of mothering skills. The case for peer support for early labour has not been explored formally. Companionship, emotional and informational support may be provided by doulas but in the UK, apart from a small number of volunteer doula services targeting support at disadvantaged women, these often require direct payment by the woman and are not routinely available. In some units, maternity support workers may be involved in supporting women in the earlier stages of labour (Sandall et al., 2006). In such settings, this appears generally to be a local arrangement that has not been formally evaluated but that is considered helpful to the organization. Owing to the widespread shortage of midwifery staff and demographic challenges within the midwifery workforce, further research is required to evaluate the feasibility and acceptability of peer or non-professional support in early labour.

Conclusions

This chapter has focused on maternity care in developed country settings where women have access to an appropriately trained healthcare professional for established labour and birth. However, it is important that the needs of women in different and less well-resourced settings are not overlooked. In such contexts, recognition of the latent phase is vitally important for women who may need to travel considerable distances to access skilled attendance for their labour and giving birth. For those women, who may be in poorer general health during pregnancy, delay in accessing skilled care is a significant contributor to maternal and neonatal death (Calvello et al., 2015). Travel to maternity facilities or trained attendants may be hazardous due to poor roads, civil unrest or a lack of accessible and affordable transport. It is important that participatory research is carried out in those settings to support women's timely and safe access to services.

Despite best intentions, currently services do not always meet women's needs regarding the advice and support they need, assessment of their labour and its progress, and care that addresses their individual circumstances. These considerations should also encompass everyone involved at this time, whether family, friends, healthcare professionals or peer supporters. Further research should take into account the constraints of service identified above and also the range of options for place of birth to which women are entitled. A number of options merit further exploration, including those outlined above. But it is important to remember that to provide optimal care, healthcare systems may need to change, rather than working from an assumption that all of the change should be expected of women and their families. A good start to labour achieved through excellent care in the latent phase will benefit women, their babies and families, and those providing maternity care. Investment in terms of high-quality, empirical research and the development of evidence-based and well-evaluated maternity services should be a priority for service providers, commissioners and users, and anyone else involved in and affected by maternity care – and is a key step to avoiding complicated latent labour, however defined.

Practice points

Organization of services

- Does your organization collect information related to service needs for latent phase labour?
- Are changes to services for latent phase labour accompanied by evaluation?
- Does your service factor in sufficient time and resources to respond to women's early labour telephone calls?

Content of care

- Does the antenatal education provided by your organization incorporate information about the latent phase? Is that information available to women and their birth companions?
- Have you considered offering a midwifery home visit during latent phase labour?
- Is your telephone advice to women in latent phase labour evidence-based and individualized to the woman's unique circumstances?
- In early labour telephone conversations, midwives should adopt a warm and confident manner, the advice offered should be clear, a rationale provided and next steps discussed; women should feel welcome to attend the maternity unit.
- Have you considered a 'call back' for women who have made contact with their birth unit in the latent phase?
- Do you encourage women to continue to use their coping strategies at times of transition, such as when transferring from home to the maternity unit in labour?

References

American College of Obstetricians and Gynecologists (ACOG) (2014) *Safe Prevention of the Primary Cesarean Delivery*. Washington, DC: American College of Obstetrics and Gynecology.

Barnett, C., Hundley, V., Cheyne, H. and Kane, F. (2008) 'Not in labour': impact of sending women home in latent phase, *British Journal of Midwifery*, 16 (3): 144–53.

Calvello, E., Skog, A.P., Tenner, A.G. and Wallis, L.A. (2015) Applying the lessons of maternal mortality reduction to global emergency health, *Bulletin of the World Health Organisation*, 93 (6): 417–23.

Carlsson, I.M., Halberg, L.R.M. and Odberg Peterssen, K. (2009) Swedish women's experiences of seeking care and being admitted during the latent phase of labour: a grounded theory study, *Midwifery*, 25 (2): 172–80.

Cheyne, H., Dowding, D.W. and Hundley, V. (2006) Making the diagnosis of labour: midwives' diagnostic judgement and management decisions, *Journal of Advanced Nursing*, 53 (6): 625–35.

Cheyne, H., Hundley, V., Dowding, D., Bland, M., McNamee, P., Greer, I. et al. (2008) Effects of algorithm for diagnosis of active labour: cluster randomised trial, *British Medical Journal*, 337: a2396.

Commission for Health Improvement (CHI) (2004) What CHI has found, in *NHS Direct Services*. London: CHI.

Dixon, L., Skinner, J. and Foureur, M. (2013) Women's perspectives of the stages and phases of labour, *Midwifery*, 29 (1): 10–17.

Dixon-Woods, M., Cavers, D., Agarwal, S., Annandale, E., Arthur, A., Harvey, J. et al. (2006) Conducting a critical interpretive synthesis of the literature on access to healthcare by vulnerable groups, *BMC Medical Research Methodology*, 6: 35.

Eri, T.S., Blystad, A., Gjengedal, E. and Blaaka, G. (2010) Negotiating credibility: first-time mothers' experiences of contact with the labour ward before hospitalisation, *Midwifery*, 26 (6): e25–30.

Ferguson, P. (2004) The pathway to normal labour, *Practising Midwife*, 7: 4–5.

Finlayson, K., Downe, S., Hinder, S., Carr, H., Spiby, H. and Whorwell, P. (2015) Unexpected consequences: women's experiences of a self-hypnosis intervention to help with pain relief during labour, *BMC Pregnancy and Childbirth*, 15: 229.

Flint, C. (1993) *Midwifery Teams and Caseloads*. Oxford: Butterworth-Heinemann.

Flint, C. (1996) Home assessment in early labour, *MIDIRS Midwifery Digest*, 6: 169–70.

Green, J.M., Spiby, H., Hucknall, C. and Richardson Foster, H. (2012) Converting policy into care: women's satisfaction with the early labour telephone component of the All Wales Clinical Pathway for Normal Labour, *Journal of Advanced Nursing*, 68 (10): 2218–28.

Gross, M.M., Haunschild, T., Stoexen, T., Methner, V. and Guenter, H.H. (2003) Women's recognition of the spontaneous onset of labor, *Birth*, 30 (4): 267–71.

Gross, M.M., Burian, R.A., Frömke, C., Hecker, H., Schippert, C. and Hillemanns, P. (2009) Onset of labour: women's experiences and midwives' assessments in relation to first stage duration, *Archives of Gynecology and Obstetrics*, 280 (6): 899–905.

Hanley, G.E., Munro, S., Greyson, D., Gross, M.M., Hundley, V., Spiby, H. et al. (2015) Onset of labour: a systematic review of definitions in the research literature, in *Collated Abstracts, Normal Labour and Birth* – 10th Research Conference, University of Central Lancashire, UK.

Hannah, M.E., Ohlsson, A., Farine, D., Hewson, S.A., Hodnett, E.D., Myhr, T.L. et al. (1996) Induction of labor compared with expectant management for prelabor rupture of the membranes at term, *New England Journal of Medicine*, 334 (16): 1005–10.

Hemminki, E. and Simukka, R. (1986) The timing of hospital admission and progress of labour, *European Journal of Obstetrics, Gynecology and Reproductive Biology*, 22 (1/2): 85–94.

Holmes, P., Oppenheimer, L.W. and Wen, S. (2001) The relationship between cervical dilatation at initial presentation in labour and subsequent intervention, *BJOG: An International Journal of Obstetrics and Gynaecology*, 108 (11): 1120–4.

Hunt, S.C. and Symonds, A. (1995) *The Social Meaning of Midwifery*. Basingstoke: Macmillan.

Janssen, P.A., Iker, C.E. and Carty, E.A. (2003) Early labour assessment and support at home: a randomized controlled trial, *Journal of Obstetrics and Gynecology*, 25 (9): 734–41.

Klein, M., Lloyd, I., Redman, C., (1983) A comparison of low risk pregnant women booked for delivery in two systems of care: shared care (consultant) and integrated general practice unit. II. Labour and delivery management and neonatal outcome, *British Journal of Obstetrics and Gynaecology*, 90 (2): 123–8.

Martin, C.R. and Jomeen, J. (2004) The impact of clinical management type on maternal locus of control in pregnant women with pre-labour rupture of membranes at term, *Human Psychology Update*, 13: 3–13.

McNiven, P.S., Williams, J.I., Hodnett, E., Kaufman, K. and Hannah, M.E. (1998) Early labour assessment improved several intrapartum outcomes, *Birth*, 25 (1): 5–10.

National Institute for Health and Clinical Excellence (NICE) (2014) *Intrapartum Care for Healthy Women and Babies*, Clinical Guideline CG190. London: NICE [https://www.nice.org.uk/guidance/cg190].

Nolan, M. (2009) Labor isn't happening until health professionals tell you so, in Roundtable Discussion: Early Labor: What's the problem?, *Birth*, 36: 332–9.

Nott, M. and Pragnell, V. (2015) '24 hour labour line': improving experiences for women, birth partners and services, in *Collated Abstracts, Normal Labour and Birth* – 10th Research Conference, University of Central Lancashire, UK.

Sandall, J., Manthorpe, J., Mansfield, A. and Spencer, L. (2006) *Support Workers in Maternity Services: A national scoping study of NHS Trusts providing maternity care in England 2006*. London: King's College, University of London.

Spiby, H., Green, J.M., Hucknall, C., Richardson Foster, H. and Andrews, A. (2007) *Labouring to Better Effect: Studies of services for women in early labour – The OPAL study (OPtions for Assessment in early Labour)*. London: HMSO.

Spiby, H., Green, J.M., Renfrew, M.J., Crawshaw, S., Stewart, P., Lishman, J. et al. (2008) *Improving Care at the Primary/Secondary Interface: A trial of community-based support in early labour – The ELSA trial*. London: HMSO.

Spiby, H., Green, J.M., Richardson-Foster, H. and Hucknall, C. (2013) Early labour services: changes, triggers, monitoring and evaluation, *Midwifery*, 29 (4): 277–83.

Spiby, H., Slade, P., Escott, D., Henderson, B. and Fraser, R.B. (2003) Selected coping strategies in labour: an investigation of women's experiences, *Birth*, 30 (3): 189–94.

Spiby, H., Walsh, D., Green, J., Crompton, A. and Bugg, G. (2014) Midwives' beliefs and concerns about telephone conversations with women in early labour, *Midwifery*, 30 (9): 1036–42.

Spiby, H., Watts, K., Stewart, J. et al. (2015) Preparation for labour and birth; the needs, preferences and experiences of first-time mothers, in *Collated Abstracts, Normal Labour and Birth* – 10th Research Conference, University of Central Lancashire, UK.

Walsh, D. (2006) Subverting the assembly-line: childbirth in a free-standing birth centre, *Social Science and Medicine*, 62 (6): 1330–40.

Weavers, A. and Nash, K., (2012) Setting up a triage telephone line for women in early labour, *British Journal of Midwifery*, 20 (5): 333–8.

Wiklund, I., Mattheison, A.-S., Klang, B. and Ransjö-Arvidson, A.-B. (2002) A comparative study in Stockholm, Sweden, of labour outcome and women's perceptions of being referred in labour, *Midwifery*, 18 (3): 193–9.

7

Maternal obesity

Angela Kerrigan

Introduction

Obesity in pregnancy is associated with a number of risks and complications, both to the mother and the fetus/neonate. The rise in the number of women who are obese during pregnancy has led to the development of national guidance for the management of this population. This chapter will focus on obesity during pregnancy and childbirth. It will aim to define obesity and outline the underlying physiology of the condition. It will look in detail at obesity in relation to pregnancy and childbearing, highlighting the rates of obesity in pregnancy globally, presenting the relevant literature about obesity in pregnancy, including the risks and challenges the condition presents. It will present the current evidence and guidance that underpin midwifery practice in relation to the management of obese, pregnant women, including examples of current midwifery practices, illustrated with real cases and examples of good practice. Finally, five key points and suggestions for further reading are provided.

What is obesity?

Medically, obesity can be viewed as a disease or, in a social context, as an increasing social trend. Tiran (2012) defines obesity as the excessive development of fat throughout the body, or an increase in weight beyond that considered desirable for an age, height and bone structure, and suggests it can affect both physical and mental wellbeing. It is further defined as the point when excess weight may seriously endanger health (Department of Health, 2008). Body mass index (BMI) is used to measure obesity and is defined as the ratio of body weight in kilograms, divided by the square of height in metres (WHO, 2000). It is usual to express BMI as a number. A desirable BMI is between 19 and 24.9 and is considered a healthy weight. A BMI between 25 and 29.9 is considered overweight, with obesity represented by a BMI above 30 (NICE, 2014a). Body mass indices above 30 have been further classified, with a BMI of 30–34.9 defined as obesity level one, 35–39.9 obesity level two and a BMI of 40 or more obesity level three (NICE, 2014a).

Obesity has reached epidemic proportions globally, with its prevalence having trebled in the UK since the 1980s (Department of Health, 2004). Currently, approximately 24% of adults are obese in the UK, with rates varying throughout the world. The highest rates of obesity are currently seen in the United States and the United Arab Emirates, with the lowest rates in China. It is estimated that, based on current trends, half of the population of the UK could be obese by 2030 (NHS Choices, 2013).

Obesity is a major public health concern because of its direct contribution to chronic diseases, such as diabetes mellitus, hypertension, high blood cholesterol, coronary heart disease, strokes and cancer (Sheiner et al., 2004). The World Health Organization consultation in 1997 (WHO, 1997) predicted obesity would become such a major public health issue in the coming decade that they called for governments all over the world to tackle the growing problem. Governments were urged to develop new preventive and therapeutic public health strategies that would affect society as a whole and would encourage weight management through dietary modifications, physical activity and lifestyle changes. However, it could be argued that these strategies have failed to prevent an obesity epidemic, as more than a decade later obesity rates worldwide are at their highest and continuing to rise and contribute to both morbidity and mortality rates.

Why is obesity in pregnancy important?

As obesity increases, so does the number of women of reproductive age who are obese. In the UK, obesity affects one-fifth of the female population (Lashen et al., 2004). The former Centre for Maternal and Child Enquiries (CMACE) considered all deaths of women during pregnancy and up to a year following childbirth. In 2011, CMACE placed a great emphasis on the effects that maternal obesity can have on pregnancy and childbearing and suggested that obesity could be one of the greatest threats to the childbearing population of the UK (CMACE, 2011).

Associated risks of obesity in pregnancy

Obesity in pregnancy has been widely researched and the literature clearly demonstrates that obese pregnant women have a higher risk of a number of pregnancy complications, including miscarriage, pre-eclampsia, gestational diabetes, fetal macrosomia and stillbirth (Kumari, 2001; Sebire et al., 2001; Stephansson et al., 2001; Cedergren, 2004; Kristensen et al., 2005; Nohr et al., 2005; Robinson et al., 2005; Heude et al., 2011; Scott-Pillai et al., 2013).

Obese woman are also at increased risk of a number of complications that arise during the intrapartum and early postnatal periods. The risk of induction of labour is reported to be double for obese pregnant women (Kiran et al., 2005; Denison et al., 2008; Arrowsmith et al., 2011). However, it could be argued that the increased incidence of pre-eclampsia and gestational diabetes greatly influences the need for induction of labour in many obese pregnant women. Nevertheless, Denison et al. (2008) and Arrowsmith et al. (2011) report increased rates of post-term pregnancy and decreased rates of spontaneous labour at term among women with a BMI above 30, which necessitate labour to be induced. Furthermore, Arrowsmith et al. (2011) also report a significant increase in the number of obese women having an emergency caesarean section following induction of labour, compared with women of normal weight.

Delay during the first stage of labour is another common complication of labour in obese women (Vahratian et al., 2004; Zhang et al., 2007; Kerrigan and Kingdon, 2010; Bogaerts et al., 2013), with the increased risk varying from 1.5 times to three times more likely. Vahratian et al. (2004) not only state that obese women have an increased risk of delay during the first stage of labour that results in caesarean section, but they also report a significantly longer length of first stage in obese women who achieve a vaginal birth. The length of labour for obese women was found to be almost two hours longer than in women of normal weight. Zhang et al. (2007) provide support for these findings and suggest inadequate uterine contractions to be the most likely reason for this, as they found a decrease in the force and frequency of contractions in obese women. Dietz et al. (2005) suggest that although the biological pathway through which obesity affects the labour process is not well understood, an increase in pelvic soft tissue may influence labour dystocia.

Obese women also have a significantly increased risk of caesarean section (Kaiser and Kirby, 2001; Sheiner et al., 2004; Dempsey et al., 2005; Kiran et al., 2005; Chu et al., 2007; Zhang et al., 2007; Kerrigan and Kingdon, 2010; Scott-Pillai et al., 2013). The increased risk of caesarean section among obese women compared with non-obese women varies from two-fold to more than three-fold, with the most common reason for caesarean section in an obese woman being delay during the first stage of labour. This delay has been shown to occur even after augmentation with oxytocin (Vahratian et al., 2004; Zhang et al., 2007; Kerrigan and Kingdon, 2010). This increased risk of caesarean section also has a considerable impact on postnatal morbidity. In a retrospective study of 611 post-operative women, maternal obesity was shown as an independent risk factor for post-caesarean infectious morbidity, regardless of whether the caesarean section was elective or emergency (Myles et al., 2002).

Shoulder dystocia is one complication of birth in obese women for which the evidence is inconsistent. Kiran et al. (2005) report that obese women with a BMI of 30 or above are four times more likely to experience shoulder dystocia during the birth of their babies. Similarly, Cedergren (2004) reported that shoulder dystocia was three times more likely in women with a BMI of 40 or above, compared with women with a normal BMI. In contrast, Kerrigan and Kingdon (2010) and Scott-Pillai et al. (2013) reported that the incidence of shoulder dystocia was not significantly higher in obese than non-obese women. In their study of the relationship between maternal obesity and shoulder dystocia, Robinson et al. (2003) concluded that maternal obesity alone is not an independent risk factor for shoulder dystocia; it is the presence of fetal macrosomia that is the most powerful indicator.

The qualitative literature on obesity and pregnancy is more limited, but studies in recent years have reported that midwives find caring for obese women during labour challenging, especially the loss of 'normality' and the challenge of promoting active labour in a medicalized birth environment (Kerrigan et al., 2015). Many midwives reported a 'heart-sinking feeling' at the prospect of looking after an obese woman in labour, because of the physical difficulties involved in providing care (Singleton and Furber, 2014). Obese pregnant women themselves report experiencing feelings of guilt when attending for maternity care, with many reporting prejudice and negative attitudes from staff because of their physical size (Nyman et al., 2008; Mulherin et al., 2013). A study looking at obese women's understanding of the associated risks of obesity in pregnancy reported that although the women were aware that obesity was a risk factor during pregnancy, they were not aware of what the risks were, with many only gaining this information during pregnancy, which led to increased anxiety throughout their pregnancy (Keely et al., 2011).

Guidance on obesity in pregnancy

In 2010, two national guidelines were published that focused on weight management and obesity during pregnancy (NICE, 2010; CMACE/RCOG, 2010). The NICE guidance on weight management during pregnancy states that being obese at the start of pregnancy will have a greater influence on both maternal and fetal health than the amount of weight a woman gains during pregnancy. However, calorie-controlled dieting is not recommended during pregnancy, as it may harm the fetus and health professionals should advise that a healthy diet and being physically active will benefit both the pregnant woman and her unborn baby. Health professionals should provide sound information on what constitutes a healthy, balanced diet and provide specific and practical advice about physical activity during pregnancy. Finally, the guidance states that support should also be provided to enable obese women to achieve a healthy weight following childbirth (NICE, 2010).

Guidance from CMACE and RCOG (2010) on the management of women with obesity in pregnancy specifically focuses on the obstetric and midwifery management of obese women during pregnancy. It suggests that the antenatal care of obese women should include consultations with both obstetricians and anaesthetists, and there should be increased surveillance for pre-eclampsia during the third trimester and a need for obese women to have a glucose tolerance test at least once during pregnancy. The guidance relating to labour and birth states that women with a BMI above 35 should give birth in a consultant-led unit and be informed of the potential complications of obesity prior to labour. It recommends that an anaesthetist be informed at the time of admission of any woman with a BMI above 40 and the early siting of an epidural may be beneficial in some circumstances. It does, however, state that obesity alone is not an indication for induction of labour, and spontaneous labour should be encouraged in the absence of any other risk factors. It is recommended that obese women should receive continuous midwifery care during labour and midwives should be vigilant in order to ensure normal labour progress. The need for continuous fetal monitoring during labour is not explicitly stated, only that the monitoring of the fetal heart can be challenging and close surveillance is required, using a fetal scalp electrode if necessary (CMACE/RCOG, 2010).

Midwifery practice for intrapartum care of obese women

The guidance surrounding the management of labour and birth in obese women is currently focused primarily on obstetric care, as is evident in the guidance on management of women with obesity in pregnancy (CMACE/RCOG, 2010), with very little reference made to midwifery care during the intrapartum period. Acknowledging the risks associated with obesity during labour and birth are key to a midwife's practice, but they must have the confidence to support women during labour and birth and promote normality, in order to optimize the chance of normal birth.

Mobility and upright positioning

'Alternative positions', those seen as any position where the woman is not semi-recumbent, including kneeling, squatting and standing, have been widely researched in relation to labour progress and birth outcomes. Midwives have a significant influence on the position adopted by labouring women and with the increasing medicalized trend to childbirth, women are expected to be more passive and compliant to the wishes of the midwife, often allowing them easy access to the emerging fetal head and perineum (Deakin, 2001). There is, however, a vast amount of evidence demonstrating the numerous benefits of upright positions and mobility during labour and birth. De Jong et al. (1997) concluded that when labouring women adopt a more upright position for labour, they experience less pain, less perineal trauma and fewer episiotomies. Adopting an upright position during labour and remaining mobile can reduce the risk of delay during the first stage of labour, decrease the total length of labour and maintain fetal and maternal wellbeing during labour (Lawrence et al., 2009; Cotton, 2010). Other advantages of upright positions in labour include: the gravitational effects on fetal descent, increased pelvic diameters, more efficient and effective uterine activity, and improved fetal alignment in the pelvis (MIDIRS, 2008). When considering the evidence on maternal position, it is difficult to understand why the adoption of a semi-recumbent position has become widely accepted practice. In contrast to alternative positions, there is little evidence to support this practice and midwives are encouraged to examine their practice in relation to this.

The decreased incidence of mobility during labour in obese women is commonly attributed to the perceived need for continuous fetal monitoring (Swann and Davis, 2012; Singleton and Furber, 2014; Kerrigan et al., 2015), but when considering the increased risk of delay during labour and the increased incidence of emergency caesarean section in obese women, it is essential that midwives promote mobility and actively encourage and assist obese women to adopt upright positions in order to minimize these risks and optimize the chance of a normal birth. As long as the fetal heart can be monitored effectively, alternative positions can be adopted and should be encouraged. Giving birth in an upright position can also minimize the risk of shoulder dystocia because of the increased pelvic diameters (Sutton, 2001). As highlighted earlier, fetal macrosomia is more common among obese women (Kumari, 2001) and is strongly associated with a higher incidence of shoulder dystocia (Robinson et al., 2003). Therefore, when fetal macrosomia is suspected, encouraging and facilitating an obese woman to birth in an upright position may significantly reduce the risk of shoulder dystocia. The promotion and facilitation of mobility are an important aspect of the role of the midwife in intrapartum care, but it could be viewed as even more important when caring for women who are at increased risk of complications during labour and birth from the outset. It is essential that midwives challenge current practices and think of alternative ways in which to support obese women to remain active and mobile during labour, while also ensuring fetal and maternal wellbeing, in order to minimize the impact of obesity on labour outcomes and maximize the opportunity for normal labour and birth.

Reflection point

How many obese women in your local unit give birth in alternative positions? What changes to your own personal practice could you make to encourage obese women to remain mobile during labour and birth?

Hydrotherapy and water birth

Using water as a form of analgesia for pain during childbirth is widely adopted across the world, with the benefits of labouring in water well documented. The Department of Health, in *Maternity Matters* (Department of Health, 2007), suggested that immersion in water should be offered to all women as a form of analgesia during labour. The physiological benefits of hydrotherapy during labour facilitate mobility and a change in maternal position and increase buoyancy (Campbell, 2004). Hydrotherapy also allows a feeling of weightlessness through the increased buoyancy, allowing women the ability and confidence to adopt upright positions, which not only increase the dimensions of the pelvic outlet, but also use gravitational forces to aid fetal descent (Sutton, 2001).

It could be argued that the use of hydrotherapy may be even more beneficial for obese women, as it may give them the confidence to mobilize during labour and adopt upright positions, which they may not otherwise have done. This is because of the increased buoyancy and sense of weightlessness they experience while in the water. This may help minimize the risk of delay during the first stage of labour, which is much more common among obese women. Swann and Davis (2012) suggest that the advantages of hydrotherapy for obese women may outweigh the disadvantages because of the potential benefits it can have for optimizing the chance of normal birth. The use of waterproof, wireless telemetry may overcome difficulties when monitoring the fetal heart and with its availability increasing, it may mean that more obese women are able to utilize hydrotherapy for both labour and birth, allowing mobility and the adoption of upright positions, while also ensuring fetal wellbeing.

Practice point

What is the guidance in your local unit on the use of hydrotherapy and water birth for obese women? Would you have the confidence to support an obese woman who wishes to labour in water?

Place of birth and birth environment

The Birthplace in England study was conducted in order to compare intrapartum and early neonatal mortality and morbidity and interventions in labour by planned place of birth for women considered at 'low risk' (Birthplace in England Collaborative Group, 2011). It demonstrated that there was no difference in the incidence of neonatal morbidity or mortality in women who planned to give birth in a midwifery-led setting, compared with an obstetric setting, regardless of parity. The exception was for nulliparous women who planned to give birth at home, where the incidence of neonatal mortality or morbidity was higher. Furthermore, interventions during labour were substantially lower in all non-obstetric settings.

A secondary analysis of the data from the study looked at the impact that maternal BMI had on intrapartum interventions and outcomes. The focus was on healthy, pregnant women, with the only risk factor being a BMI of 35 or above. The findings supported the evidence presented earlier in the chapter, showing that maternal obesity is associated with increased risks of adverse intrapartum outcomes. Otherwise healthy obese women have an increased risk of augmentation, intrapartum caesarean section and some adverse maternal outcomes, but the increased risk was described as 'modest'. Interestingly, it demonstrated that multiparous obese women with no additional risk factors are at lower risk of requiring obstetric care during labour and birth compared with 'low-risk' nulliparous women of normal weight. It was therefore concluded that BMI should be considered in conjunction with parity when assessing the potential risks associated with birth in non-obstetric unit settings (Hollowell et al., 2014).

The guidance from CMACE and RCOG (2010) states that women with a BMI of 35 or above should give birth in a consultant-led obstetric unit, with access to neonatal services because women with obesity are at significantly higher risk of intrapartum complications. Although the NICE guidance on intrapartum care (NICE, 2014b) recommends that women with a BMI of 35 or above should be advised to give birth in an obstetric unit in order to reduce the risk of adverse outcomes in both the mother and the fetus/neonate, it reflects the findings of the Birthplace in England study (Hollowell et al., 2014) and now states that women who have a BMI of 30–35 at booking should have an individualized assessment and discussion during pregnancy, regarding their choice of place of birth, with midwifery-led settings not ruled out.

A safe and comfortable birth environment facilitates the release of labour hormones and facilitates effective uterine activity in order to allow labour to progress effectively (Buckley, 2004). Page (2000) suggests that women should be able to labour in a protected environment where they are able to cope with labour and feel safe. A very clinical or technological environment may cause anxiety or apprehension, which could adversely affect labour progress (Enkin et al., 2000). Although the guidance on obesity in pregnancy (CMACE/RCOG, 2010) recommends that obese women with a BMI of 35 or above should give birth in an obstetric unit, midwives should have the confidence to challenge this practice when taking into account other factors, such as parity and whether an alternative place of birth (e.g. a midwifery-led unit) may be more appropriate. However, obese women who choose to give birth in an obstetric unit should still be able to labour in a comfortable, calm and private environment in order to maximize the release of labour hormones, stimulate effective uterine contractions and minimize the risk of labour becoming prolonged. Midwives can achieve this by employing simple strategies, such as ensuring privacy, making the room comfortable and homely, and dimming the lights. Changing the arrangement of the furniture, so that the bed is not the focus of the room, is another easy way to make a birthing room more comfortable and welcoming. Providing alternative 'furniture' in the form or beanbags or birthing balls makes a birthing environment more comfortable, while simultaneously facilitating mobility and upright positioning. These strategies should still be employed when caring for an obese woman in labour, even if there is a need to perform continuous fetal monitoring, as this can still be performed through careful positioning of equipment. These simple strategies will increase normality for obese women during labour and birth and optimize the chance of a normal birth.

Reflection point

What is the birth environment like for obese women in your local unit? How could you adapt this to encourage normality?

The national guidance does, however, recommend that women with a BMI of 40 or above should receive continuous support from a midwife during labour and birth (CMACE/RCOG, 2010). Continuous midwifery care is recommended for all women in established labour, but it is suggested that midwives need to be more vigilant to ensure normal labour progress in women with a BMI of 40 or above, which can be facilitated by a constant midwifery presence during labour. Hodnett et al. (2011) suggest that continuous support during labour and birth reduces both the length of labour and the rate of caesarean section, and has a direct impact on women's experience of childbirth. Sandall (2004) reports that women who have continuous support during labour are more likely to have a normal birth and less likely to need intrapartum analgesia. Supporting a woman during labour, however, does not just mean being physically present in the room, but also involves providing both physical and emotional support (Enkin et al., 2000). However, Hodnett et al. (2011) suggest that this support does not necessarily have to be provided by a midwife, and women may in fact benefit more from support from a person who is not providing care simultaneously. Enkin et al. (2000) advocate that every woman should be able to choose who should provide support during labour, which ought to be based on who is the most appropriate and effective person for this role. Obese women have significantly increased risks of prolonged labour and caesarean section, and therefore it could be argued that these women should be prioritized for continuous midwifery care during labour, acknowledging the national guidance, in order to ensure labour progresses effectively – and that the chance of normal birth is maximized. Obese women should also be informed, before the onset of labour, of the importance of good support during labour and birth, and they should be encouraged to choose a birth partner who will provide both effective and constant physical and emotional support for them throughout their labour.

Case 7.1: Local guidance

In one NHS maternity unit, the local guidance on the care of women with a BMI of 35 or above has been adapted to reflect the needs of the local population and the wishes of women. The inclusion criteria for giving birth on the neighbouring midwifery-led unit (MLU) have been increased, to include women with a BMI up to and including 39.9. The multidisciplinary team made this decision after many obese women, particularly multiparous women, expressed their desire to give birth on the MLU and use hydrotherapy. While acknowledging the national guidance and the increased intrapartum risks associated with obesity, it was felt that increasing the inclusion criteria for admission to the MLU would enable more obese women to experience 'normal' labour and maximize their chance of normal birth. Regular audits of perinatal outcomes are carried out in order to ensure safety, with the option to review the guideline if indicated. This practice reflects the findings of the Birthplace in England study (Hollowell et al., 2014), which focused on healthy, pregnant women with a BMI of 35 and concluded that BMI should be considered in conjunction with parity when assessing the potential risks of giving birth in midwifery-led settings.

Multidisciplinary care

The national guidance on obesity in pregnancy recommends that the management of women with obesity in pregnancy should be integrated into all antenatal clinics, with clear policies and guidelines for care available. Specialist antenatal services are available in some hospitals across the UK, although specialist clinics are not feasible in all areas, particularly those with a high prevalence of obesity because of resource limitations (CMACE/RCOG, 2010). All health professionals providing care to obese women during pregnancy should be aware of the risks associated with maternal obesity. It is also recommended that women with a booking BMI of 30 or above should be informed during their pregnancy about the possible complications during labour and birth that are associated with a high BMI. It is recommended that women should be referred to a consultant obstetrician to enable this discussion (CMACE/RCOG, 2010), although, with appropriate education, it could be argued that midwives would be able to have this discussion with women and it could be viewed as an opportunity to formulate a birth plan that acknowledges the associated risks of obesity, reflects the wishes of the woman and promotes normality during labour and birth. Additionally, pregnant women with a BMI of 40 or above should have a consultation with an obstetric anaesthetist during the antenatal period, in order to discuss an anaesthetic management plan, should it become necessary during the intrapartum period, while also assessing any potential difficulties with regional or general anaesthesia (CMACE/RCOG, 2010).

A shared-care approach to antenatal care is recommended for all obese women, and although the recommendations state that obese pregnant women should have consultations during the antenatal period with obstetricians and anaesthetists, it is essential that midwives are also involved in the care of obese women. Every pregnant woman has the opportunity to make choices about the maternity care she receives, including the type of antenatal care (Department of Health, 2007), so it is therefore essential to educate obese pregnant women why shared care is considered to be the safest and most appropriate form of care and an individualized plan of care should be outlined (Department of Health, 2007). Midwives play a vital role in the care of obese women, in order to meet her social, emotional and educational needs, thus each woman should have regular contact with a midwife, regardless of who her lead care provider is (Kerrigan and Kingdon, 2010).

Informing women and discussing the potential complications during labour and birth should be done in a way that will educate and empower women to minimize these risks during the intrapartum period. It should not be done in a way that might increase anxiety and cause women to feel that they will not be able to experience normal birth. The Nursing and Midwifery Council (NMC, 2012: 7) state: 'You should make sure the needs of the woman and her baby are the primary focus of your practice and you should work in partnership with the woman and her family, providing safe, responsive, compassionate care in an appropriate environment to facilitate her physical and emotional care throughout childbirth.' Ensuring obese women are fully informed of the risks associated with obesity during labour and birth will equip them with the knowledge they require in order to identify strategies that they could employ during labour and birth that will optimize their chance of normal birth, feel in control during labour and give them a positive childbirth experience. CMACE and RCOG (2010) recommend that in addition to providing women with information on the associated risks, they should also have the opportunity to discuss how these risks could be minimized; therefore midwives, with the appropriate education and knowledge, play a key role in the education and empowerment of obese women in their preparation for labour and birth.

Following an informed discussion about the potential complications during labour and birth, each woman should have the opportunity to formulate a birth plan that reflects her wishes, promotes normality and encourages normal birth. A birth plan is a plan that records a woman's preferences for labour and birth, which is prepared by the woman in collaboration with her partner and her midwife (Tiran, 2012). The formulation of birth plans for obese women may involve the wider multidisciplinary team, in order to ensure safety of both the mother and the fetus/neonate. This is particularly important if the wishes of the woman are outside of the recommendations of the local and national guidance. In addition to midwives, obstetricians and anaesthetists, Supervisors of midwives play a key role in the process of birth planning for 'high-risk' women. The roles and responsibilities of Supervisors of midwives are wide and varied and in addition to protecting mothers and babies and ensuring safe standards of midwifery practice (NMC, 2009), they play a key role in promoting childbirth as a normal, physiological event, being an advocate for women to allow them to make informed choices and providing support to midwives who are supporting women in making choices about their care (NMC, 2010). Supervisors of midwives are therefore ideally placed to contribute to the formulation of birth plans for obese women and should be seen as a key part of the team. The involvement of a Supervisor of midwives in the birth planning for an obese woman ensures she can make informed choices about her care, ensures safety of both the woman and her baby, while acknowledging the associated risks, ensures a positive experience and maximizes the chance of normal labour and birth. Communication is key to this and should occur across all disciplines, with the woman and her family at the centre.

Case 7.2: Jennifer

Jennifer was G2P1, with a booking BMI of 43. She had had a normal birth with her son two years previously, with no intrapartum or postnatal complications. Jennifer had attended for antenatal care regularly and at 28 weeks had met with the consultant obstetrician who had informed her of the associated risks of obesity during labour and birth. He advised that in view of her increased risk of prolonged labour and increased likelihood of caesarean section, she should give birth in the delivery suite at the consultant-led unit. Jennifer was disappointed with this, as she had previously experienced a normal labour and birth and wished to give birth in the neighbouring midwifery-led unit.

At her next appointment with the community midwife, Jennifer expressed her disappointment and anxiety at having to give birth in the consultant-led delivery suite. The midwife spoke to Jennifer about the increased risks associated with obesity and informed her of strategies that she could employ in order to reduce these risks. The midwife spoke about the importance of remaining mobile during her labour, adopting upright positions and the option of hydrotherapy as a form of analgesia. Jennifer and the midwife then devised a birth plan that reflected her wishes.

In view of the associated risks of obesity during labour and birth, the midwife liaised with the obstetrician and her own supervisor of midwives and discussed the birth plan that she and Jennifer had devised. It was felt that in view of Jennifer's history of a previous normal labour and birth and the fact she was fully informed of the risks of obesity during labour and birth, Jennifer's wish to give birth in the neighbouring midwifery-led unit should be facilitated. The midwife and the supervisor of midwives made certain that strategies were in place to ensure the safety of both Jennifer and her baby. It was agreed that Jennifer would attend the neighbouring midwifery-led unit when she was in labour and aim for a normal birth, but with the understanding that if there were any complications during her labour and/or concerns for the wellbeing of Jennifer or her baby, she would be transferred to the delivery suite.

Jennifer went into spontaneous labour at 39 + 1 weeks' gestation, and attended the neighbouring midwifery-led unit where, on admission, her cervix was 5 cm dilated. The midwife caring for her reviewed her birth plan on admission and reiterated the importance of mobility during labour and facilitated this by providing Jennifer with a birthing ball to use. Jennifer and her midwife agreed that if the midwife were concerned at any point during labour about the safety of either Jennifer or her baby, Jennifer would be transferred to the consultant-led delivery suite. Jennifer remained mobile during labour, utilized the birthing ball and had a normal birth on all fours, approximately three hours later.

Jennifer felt very positive about her birth experience as her wishes had been acknowledged and although she was aware of the associated risks of obesity, she felt empowered to aim for a normal birth, through the support she received from her community midwife, the supervisor of midwives and the midwife who cared for her during her labour. This illustrates how women who may otherwise have been excluded from a midwifery-led unit for labour and birth can have a positive birth experience through clear communication across the multidisciplinary team and also through the inclusion of a supervisor of midwives in the planning of care, ensuring safety, promoting normal birth and providing support to midwives.

Conclusion

This chapter has illustrated the impact maternal obesity can have on pregnancy and childbirth, including the increased risk of complications during labour and birth. It has described ways that midwives can encourage and facilitate normal birth when caring for obese women, including the active promotion of mobility and upright positioning, facilitating the use of hydrotherapy, ensuring the birth environment and the choice of place of birth reflect the wishes of the woman and encourage effective labour progress. Finally, it has demonstrated how, through effective multidisciplinary care and communication, the wishes of obese women can be fulfilled, culminating in a positive birth experience.

Key points

- Obesity in pregnancy is associated with a number of adverse complications during pregnancy, labour and birth, and the postnatal period.
- Midwives play a key role in 'normalizing' labour and birth for obese women and should actively encourage normality in order to optimize the chance of normal birth.
- Obese women should be supported to mobilize during labour, adopt upright positions and utilize hydrotherapy in order to reduce the risk of delay during labour and the need for caesarean section.
- A multidisciplinary team should be involved in the care of obese women during pregnancy and birth, with the woman at the centre of the care.
- National guidance and guidance from the local unit provide evidence to support the care of obese women during labour and birth, but may also be challenged and adapted to reflect the individual wishes of women.

Further reading

Centre for Maternal and Child Enquiry and Royal College of Obstetricians and Gynaecologists (2010) *Management of Women with Obesity in Pregnancy: CMACE and RCOG joint guidance.* London: CMACE and RCOG [https://www.rcog.org.uk/globalassets/documents/guidelines/cmacercogjointguidelinemanagementwomenobesitypregnancya.pdf].

Downe, S. (ed.) (2004) *Normal Childbirth: Evidence and debate.* London: Churchill Livingstone.

National Institute for Health and Clinical Excellence (NICE) (2010) *Weight Management Before, During and After Pregnancy.* Public Health Guideline PH27. London: NICE [https://www.nice.org.uk/guidance/ph27/resources/weight-management-before-during-and-after-pregnancy-1996242046405].

Rees, M., Karoshi, M.A. and Keith, L. (eds) (2008) *Obesity and Pregnancy.* London: CRC Press.

References

Arrowsmith, S., Wray, S. and Quenby, S. (2011) Maternal obesity and labour complications following induction of labour in prolonged pregnancy, *BJOG: An International Journal of Obstetrics and Gynaecology*, 118: 578–88.
Birthplace in England Collaborative Group (2011) Perinatal and maternal outcomes by planned place of birth for healthy women with low risk pregnancies: the Birthplace in England national prospective cohort study, *British Medical Journal*, 343: d7400.

Bogaerts, A., Whitters, I., Van den Bergh, B., Jans, G. and Devlieger, R. (2013) Obesity in pregnancy: altered onset and progression of labour, *Midwifery*, 29: 1303–13.

Buckley, S. (2004) Undisturbed birth: nature's hormonal blue print for safety, ease and ecstasy, *MIDIRS Midwifery Digest*, 14 (2): 203–9.

Campbell, G. (2004) Critical incident analysis of water immersion, *British Journal of Midwifery*, 12 (1): 7–11.

Cedergren, M.I. (2004) Maternal morbid obesity and the risk of adverse pregnancy outcome, *Obstetrics and Gynaecology*, 103 (2): 219–24.

Centre for Maternal and Child Enquiries (CMACE) (2011) Saving mothers' lives – Reviewing maternal deaths to make motherhood safer: 2006–2008. The Eighth Report of the confidential enquiries into maternal deaths in the United Kingdom, *BJOG: An International Journal of Obstetrics and Gynaecology*, 118 (suppl.1): 1–203.

Centre for Maternal and Child Enquiry and Royal College of Obstetricians and Gynaecologists (CMACE/RCOG) (2010) *Management of Women with Obesity in Pregnancy: CMACE and RCOG joint guidance*. London: CMACE and RCOG [https://www.rcog. org.uk/globalassets/documents/guidelines/cmacercogjointguidelinemanagement-womenobesitypregnancya.pdf].

Chu, S.Y., Kim, S.Y., Scmid, C.H., Dietz, P.M., Callaghan, W.M., Lau, J. et al. (2007) Maternal obesity and risk of caesarean delivery: a meta-analysis, *Obesity Reviews*, 8: 385–94.

Cotton, J. (2010) Considering the evidence for upright positions in labour, *MIDIRS Midwifery Digest*, 20 (4): 459–63.

Deakin, B. (2001) Alternative positions in labour and childbirth, *British Journal of Midwifery*, 9 (10): 620–5.

De Jong, P., Johansson, K., Baxen, P. (1997) Randomised trial comparing the upright and supine positions for the second stage of labour, *BJOG: An International Journal of Obstetrics and Gynaecology*, 104 (5): 567–71.

Dempsey, J.C., Ashiny, Z., Qiu, C.F., Miller, R.S., Sorensen, T.K. and Williams, M.A. (2005) Maternal pre-pregnancy overweight status and obesity as risk factors for caesarean delivery, *Journal of Maternal, Fetal and Neonatal Medicine*, 17 (3): 179–85.

Denison, F.C., Price, J., Graham, C., Wild, S. and Liston, W.A. (2008) Maternal obesity, length of gestation, risk of postdates pregnancy, and spontaneous onset of labour at term, *BJOG: An International Journal of Obstetrics and Gynaecology*, 115 (6): 720–5.

Department of Health (2004) *Summary of Intelligence on Obesity: Choosing health summaries*. London: Department of Health.

Department of Health (2007) *Maternity Matters: Choice, access and continuity of care in a safe service*. London: Department of Health.

Department of Health (2008) *Healthy Weight, Healthy Lives: A cross-government strategy for England*. London: Department of Health.

Dietz, P.M., Callaghan, W.M., Morrow, B. and Cogswell, M.E. (2005) Population-based assessment of the risk of primary caesarean delivery due to excess pre-pregnancy weight among nulliparous women delivering term infants, *Maternal and Child Health Journal*, 9 (3): 237–44.

Enkin, M., Keirse, M.J.N.C., Neilson, J., Crowther, C., Duley, L., Hodnett, E. et al. (2000) *A Guide to Effective Care in Pregnancy and Childbirth* (3rd edn). Oxford: Oxford University Press.

Heude, B., Thiebaugeorges, O., Goua, V., Forhan, A., Kaminski, M., Foliguet, B. et al. (2011) Pre-pregnancy body mass index and weight gain during pregnancy: relations with gestational diabetes and hypertension, and birth outcomes, *Maternal Child Health Journal*, 16 (2): 335–63.

Hodnett, E.D., Gates, S., Hofmeyr, G.J. and Sakala, C. (2011) Continuous support for women during childbirth *Cochrane Database of Systematic Reviews*, 2: CD003766.

Hollowell, J., Pillas, D., Rowe, R., Linsell, L., Knight, M. and Brocklehurst, P. (2014) The impact of maternal obesity on intrapartum outcomes in otherwise low risk women: a secondary analysis of the Birthplace national prospective cohort study, *BJOG: An International Journal of Obstetrics and Gynaecology*, 121 (3): 343–55.

Kaiser, P.S. and Kirby, R.S. (2001) Obesity as a risk factor for caesarean section in a low-risk population, *Obstetrics and Gynaecology*, 97 (1): 39–43.

Keely, A., Gunning, M. and Denison, F. (2011) Maternal obesity in pregnancy: women's understanding of risks, *British Journal of Midwifery*, 19 (6): 364–9.

Kerrigan, A.M. and Kingdon, C. (2010) Maternal obesity and pregnancy: a retrospective study, *Midwifery*, 26: 138–46.

Kerrigan, A., Kingdon, C. and Cheyne, H. (2015) Obesity and normal birth: a qualitative study of clinicians' management of obese pregnant women during labour, *BMC Pregnancy and Childbirth*, 15: 256.

Kiran, T.S., Hemmadi, S., Bethel, J. and Evans, J. (2005) Outcome of pregnancy in a woman with an increased body mass index, *BJOG: An International Journal of Obstetrics and Gynaecology*, 112 (6): 768–72.

Kristensen, J., Vestergaard, M., Wisborg, K., Kesmodel, U. and Secher, N.J. (2005) Pre-pregnancy weight and the risk of stillbirth and neonatal death, *British Journal of Obstetrics and Gynaecology*, 112 (4): 403–8.

Kumari, A.S. (2001) Pregnancy outcome in women with morbid obesity, *International Journal of Gynaecology and Obstetrics*, 73 (3): 101–7.

Lashen, H., Fear, K. and Sturdee, D.W. (2004) Obesity is associated with increased risk of first trimester and recurrent miscarriage: matched case-control study, *Human Reproduction*, 19 (7): 1644–6.

Lawrence, A., Lewis, L., Hofmeyr, G.J. (2009) Maternal positions and mobility during first stage of labour, *Cochrane Database of Systematic Reviews*, 2: CD003934.

Midwives Information and Resource Service (MIDIRS) (2008) *Positions in Labour.* MIDIRS informed choice leaflet. London: MIDIRS.

Mulherin, K., Miller, Y., Barlow, F., Diedrichs, P. and Thompson, R. (2013) Weight stigma in maternity care: women's attitudes, experiences and care providers' attitudes, *BMC Pregnancy and Childbirth*, 13: 19.

Myles, T.D., Gooch, J. and Santolaya, J. (2002) Obesity as an independent risk factor for infectious morbidity in patients who undergo caesarean delivery, *Obstetrics and Gynecology*, 5 (1): 959–64.

National Institute for Health and Clinical Excellence (NICE) (2010) *Weight Management Before, During and After Pregnancy.* Public Health Guideline PH27. London: NICE [https://www.nice.org.uk/guidance/ph27].

National Institute for Health and Clinical Excellence (NICE) (2014a) *Obesity: Identification, assessment and management.* Clinical Guidance CG189. London: NICE [https://www.nice.org.uk/guidance/cg189].

National Institute for Health and Clinical Excellence (NICE) (2014b) *Intrapartum Care for Healthy Women and Babies.* Clinical Guideline CG190. London: NICE [https://www.nice.org.uk/guidance/cg190].

NHS Choices (2013) *Half of UK Obese by 2030* [www.nhs.uk/news; accessed 2 October 2013].

Nohr, E.A., Bech, H., Davies, M.J., Frydenberg, M., Henriksen, T.B. and Olsen, J. (2005) Pre-pregnancy obesity and fetal death, *Obstetrics and Gynecology*, 106 (2): 250–8.

Nursing and Midwifery Council (NMC) (2009) *Modern Supervision in Action: A practical guide for midwives*. London: NMC.

Nursing and Midwifery Council (NMC) (2010) *Standards for the Preparation and Practice of Supervisors of Midwives*. London: NMC.

Nursing and Midwifery Council (NMC) (2012) *Midwives' Rules and Standards*. London: NMC [https://www.nmc.org.uk/standards/additional-standards/midwives-rules-and-standards/].

Nyman, V.M., Prebensen, A.K. and Flesner, G.E.M. (2008) Obese women's experiences of encounters with midwives and physicians during pregnancy and childbirth, *Midwifery*, 26 (4): 424–9.

Page, L. (2000) Keeping birth normal, in L. Page (ed.) *The New Midwifery*. London: Churchill Livingstone.

Robinson, H., Tkatch, S., Mayes, D.C., Bott, N. and Okun, N. (2003) Is maternal obesity a predictor of shoulder dystocia?, *Obstetrics and Gynecology*, 101 (1): 24–7.

Robinson, H.E., O'Connell, C.M., Joseph, K.S. and McLeod, N.L. (2005) Maternal outcomes in pregnancies complicated by obesity, *Obstetrics and Gynecology*, 106 (6): 1357–64.

Sandall, J. (2004) Promoting normal birth: weighing the evidence, in S. Downe (ed.) *Normal Childbirth: Evidence and debate*. London: Churchill Livingstone.

Scott-Pillai, R., Spence, D., Cardwell, C.R., Hunter, A. and Holmes, V.A. (2013) The impact of body mass index on maternal and neonatal outcomes: a retrospective study in a UK obstetric population 2004–2011, *BJOG: An International Journal of Obstetrics and Gynaecology*, 120 (8): 932–9.

Sebire, N.J., Jolly, M., Harris, J.P., Wadsworth, J., Joffe, M., Beard, R.W. et al. (2001) Maternal obesity and pregnancy outcome: a study of 287 213 pregnancies in London, *International Journal of Obesity*, 25 (8): 1175–82.

Sheiner, E., Levy, A., Menes, T.S., Silverberg, D., Katz, M. and Mazor, M. (2004) Maternal obesity as an independent risk factor of caesarean delivery, *Paediatric and Perinatal Epidemiology*, 18 (3): 196–201.

Singleton, G. and Furber, C. (2014) The experiences of midwives when caring for obese women in labour: a qualitative study, *Midwifery*, 30: 103–11.

Stephansson, O., Dickman, P., Johansson, A. and Cnattingius, S. (2001) Maternal weight, pregnancy weight gain and the risk of antepartum stillbirth, *American Journal of Obstetrics and Gynecology*, 184 (3): 463–9.

Sutton, J. (2001) *Let Birth Be Born Again: Rediscovering and reclaiming our midwifery heritage*. Bedfont: Birth Concepts UK.

Swann, L. and Davis, S. (2012) The role of the midwife in improving normal birth rates in obese women, *British Journal of Midwifery*, 20 (1): 7–12.

Tiran, D. (2012) *Ballière's Midwives' Dictionary* (12th edn.). London: Ballière Tindall.

Vahratian, A., Zhang, J., Troendle, J.F., Savitz, D.A. and Siega-Riz, A.M. (2004) Maternal prepregnancy overweight and obesity and the pattern of labour progression in term nulliparous women, *Obstetrics and Gynecology*, 104 (5: Part 1): 943–51.

World Health Organization (WHO) (1997) *Obesity: Preventing and managing the global epidemic. Report of a WHO consultation on obesity*. Geneva: WHO.

World Health Organization (WHO) (2000) *Obesity: Preventing and managing the global epidemic. Report of a WHO consultation on obesity*, WHO Technical Report Series 894). Geneva: WHO [http://www.who.int/nutrition/publications/obesity/WHO_TRS_894/en/].

Zhang, J., Bricker, L., Wray, S. and Quenby, S. (2007) Poor uterine contractility in obese women, *BJOG: An International Journal of Obstetrics and Gynaecology*, 114 (3): 343–8.

8

Breech birth

Jane Evans

Introduction

Throughout history, 3–4% of all births have been breech births (RCOG, 2006). It has always been recognized that while the majority of these breech births are quite normal and successful there are some, as with cephalic births, that are pathological and therefore require help. In the early to mid-twentieth century, as more women were choosing to birth in hospital, it was still quite normal for breech births to occur at home. A breech-presenting baby was not a criterion for a hospital birth. It was not until the Peel Report (1970), which recommended that a hospital bed should be made available to every birthing woman that most births occurred in hospital. At this time, breech birth was still considered to be unusual but normal. Over the next 30 years, breech presentation was gradually deemed to be abnormal.

In the 1980s and 1990s, the skills for attending a breech delivery were becoming quite rare as lower segment caesarean section (LSCS) increased in popularity among the obstetric population and was thought to be the safest option. Since the results of the Term Breech Trial were published (Hannah et al., 2000) and the rapid implementation of the recommendations therein, there has been little option for women whose babies were presenting breech at term but to have a LSCS. Many midwives and obstetricians had serious reservations about the conduct and findings of the study, including the methodology, ethics and inappropriate inclusions to the trial. It subsequently became one of the most severely criticized randomized controlled trials in history (Kotaska, 2004; Glezerman, 2006; Turner, 2006; Lawson, 2012).

The two-year follow-up to this trial found no statistical differences could be shown between the two intention-to-treat groups of women and babies following either a vaginal or caesarean birth (Hannah et al., 2004; Whyte et al., 2004). Sadly, the original recommendations were not rescinded even though this was called for (Glezerman, 2006).

These influences have brought obstetricians and midwives to the point of having lost the knowledge and skills required to assist a woman to give birth to her breech-presenting baby vaginally, making LSCS her only option in many areas of the world. The UK Nursing and Midwifery Council (NMC, 2009, 2012) requires every registered midwife to be competent to support a breech birth in an emergency but experience is very hard to acquire.

There is now evidence to suggest that LSCS is not necessarily the best option for all women, with raised maternal mortality rates and short- and long-term morbidity rates for neonates (Silver et al., 2006; Schutte et al., 2007; O'Neill et al., 2013). However, the evidence does appear to suggest that the breech baby – at the time of birth only – may be better off being delivered by LSCS, as some breech babies born vaginally require early resuscitation and neonatal intensive care unit (NICU) support (Hannah et al., 2000; RCOG, 2006). The longer-term outlook after a caesarean delivery shows a higher incidence of obesity, diabetes, auto-immune diseases and allergies, among other complications, for the baby delivered by LSCS (Huh et al., 2012; Darmasseelane et al., 2014; Huang et al., 2015; Sevelsted et al., 2015). LSCS is expensive and in these days of financial stricture, any unnecessary expense should be avoided wherever possible.

How can breech birth be brought back into normality?

It is now being recognized and accepted that the professions caring for parturient women need to re-learn the skills to support vaginal breech births, for the health of both mothers and babies. There are, at present, one or two areas within the UK where the midwives, obstetricians, paediatricians and management work together to provide a service for women that supports vaginal breech birth. There is discussion, support and close working conditions between the whole team – all to the benefit of the woman and baby.

A major part of our re-skilling journey is to learn and observe how a breech baby comes through the birth canal. This includes refreshing our knowledge of anatomy and physiology, including being aware of the influence of the hormones and how the hormones are influenced in labour. A calm, peaceful environment supports the physiology and enables the labour to progress well and in this context the outlook for a vaginal birth is good.

Several studies have shown that, with the appropriate skills and support, vaginal delivery is as safe as LSCS delivery (Goffinet et al., 2006; Maier et al., 2011). These studies addressed the standard breech delivery, with the mother in the lithotomy position and the baby manoeuvred. To date, there have been very few published studies of the outcome for breech babies when the mother is in an all-fours or upright position and the baby births spontaneously (Borbolla Foster et al., 2014; Bogner et al., 2015). However, a 10-year study has been published in 2016 by Louwen et al. which shows outstanding results for breech birth in an all-fours position.

Normality must include a healthy, well-grown baby. Babies who have intra-uterine growth restriction (IUGR), are small for gestational age or who have an anomaly do not fare well when attempting a spontaneous breech birth, so careful, honest antenatal care will best support the parents in their decision-making.

Antenatal care

Approximately 20% of all babies are in a breech presentation at 28 weeks gestation and by term (37–42 weeks) 3–4% are still breech (RCOG, 2006). This means that the earlier the gestation when labour starts, the higher the chance of the baby being in a breech presentation at the start of labour. Prematurity brings its own set of problems and, together with the possible complications of a breech vaginal birth, can make this a tough entrance to the world for the baby. A baby less than 36 weeks gestation has a greater head-to-buttocks ratio, so a small body can slip through a partially dilated cervix and the head could then be entrapped – the same complication can potentially occur when the baby is IUGR (Larciprete et al., 2005; RCOG, 2006). This is a different complication to those encountered by a full-term, well-grown baby whose bi-parietal and bi-trochanteric diameters are similar and who has descended in the birth canal.

Discussion, support and advice throughout pregnancy about lifestyle choices will help couples to attain a healthy pregnancy and a well-grown baby. But once a breech presentation has been identified, a practitioner who is experienced and knowledgeable about all the options for a breech-presenting baby should counsel the parents. These options include whether the baby should be encouraged to turn. If so, this can be facilitated with exercises, homoeopathy, osteopathy, moxibustion or external cephalic version (ECV). It is good practice to develop a list of complementary practitioners who have experience working with women who have a breech-presenting baby. Discussion about options for the birth should cover the whole range from spontaneous vaginal breech birth, vaginal delivery/extraction, LSCS at 38 weeks gestation, LSCS at the start of labour to LSCS if the labour does not progress and needs help.

Well-informed parents then feel supported to make the appropriate decision for themselves and their baby with confident, skilled professionals attending, whatever their decision. Some may choose to birth at home, as this is where they feel safest and most relaxed.

Case 8.1: Andrea

Andrea and James were expecting their first baby and planned a home birth. All progressed well with the pregnancy until the baby was discovered to be breech at 28 weeks gestation. Andrea tried exercises and moxibustion to encourage the baby to turn but declined ECV. They talked through their options with their midwife who had breech birth experience and chose to continue with their planned home birth.

The local hospital was willing to support a spontaneous breech birth but Andrea felt she would be more relaxed at home. A second experienced midwife was available to support Andrea, James and their midwife through the birth.

The baby palpated as right sacrum anterior (RSA) but did not engage until the start of labour. Spontaneous labour started at home and progressed well over night. Andrea followed her body's messages throughout labour and was active for some and resting at other times. She stayed well hydrated and emptied her bladder as needed. Labour progressed well and when it was observed that Andrea's cervix was fully dilated, she felt tired and lay down and fell into a deep sleep, waking only for a strong contraction every ten minutes. After 30 minutes, she woke and started to push. The second stage progressed spontaneously and soon the baby's anterior buttock was visible. The baby continued to birth spontaneously, making the movements and rotations to help her birth, and was soon passed between her mother's legs to be greeted by her parents. No resuscitation was required and the third stage was completed physiologically. Andrea's perineum was intact.

Late pregnancy

Normal practice, with a full-term, well-grown baby, indicates that labour should start spontaneously, thus avoiding induction by any means, including use of any complementary therapies, cervical sweeps or chemical induction. The hormonal changes that take place during the last few days of pregnancy prepare the woman's body for labour with the baby continuing to settle into an optimal position. Precipitating labour, in any way, before these changes have occurred may cause the birth to proceed less smoothly. If labour does not start within the normal gestation of 42 completed weeks, there may be a reason for delay and a planned LSCS may be optimal. Some women naturally have a longer gestation but also the hormonal preparations for labour might be delayed when a breech-presenting baby is diagnosed late in pregnancy and options for birth need to be reconsidered.

Breech-presenting babies, at term, present on the left in approximately 45% of cases and on the right in the other 55%. There has been no formal research on this to date.

The optimal position for the baby to enter the brim of the pelvis at the end of pregnancy, and thus for the start of labour, is right sacrum anterior (RSA) (Figure 8.1.A). This encourages the spontaneous, full rotation that brings the arms through the pelvis to birth (Evans, 2012a, 2012b).

Labour

Once spontaneous labour starts, it is imperative to support the woman in a quiet, peaceful, relaxed atmosphere, remembering the effect of adrenaline on oxytocin production (Odent, 2002) and the pelvic floor sphincters (Frye, 2010). Fear is contagious and has no place in the birthing room. A relaxed, well-supported, undisturbed woman will labour optimally. Women may be quite active in labour or they may choose to lie down. She will know what is best for her baby and this particular labour – it is best not to disturb or direct her unless there is some indication of a delay.

It is important that there is communication between the baby and the mother, so narcotics and epidural anaesthesia are not advisable pain relief for a normal breech birth. Most women receive adequate pain support from relaxation, massage, TENS and inhalation analgesia. Some women use water immersion for the first stage of labour but a planned water birth is not advised, as the water pressure and buoyancy interfere with the descent and movements the baby needs to make to be born spontaneously, although some undiagnosed breech babies are born under water!

Labour, once established, is often rapid and a well-progressing labour is optimal, although a slow labour can still result in a vaginal breech birth. Midwives who are experienced with breech birth have observed that many primigravid women give birth in 6–8 hours (the duration of an average primigravid cephalic birth is 12–14 hours).

Internal examinations should be avoided, as they are an invasive procedure and may disturb the woman, especially if she is one of the 20–40% of women who have been sexually abused (Garratt, 2011). Careful observation of the woman's behaviour will indicate that the labour is progressing. In early labour, women are generally quite chatty, before needing to concentrate through contractions, as they become closer together, stronger and longer, but are still able to communicate between them. This indicates that the cervix is about 5 cm dilated. Everyone supporting the birth may feel tired and sleepy when the cervix is about 7 cm, and when the woman's cervix is between 8 and 9 cm she may become restless, agitated and monosyllabic and generally more active. Anal dilation, the appearance of the Rhombus of Michaelis and the purple line that progresses up the anal cleft of some women (see Chapter 12) will indicate full dilatation once it reaches the sacral-coccygeal joint (Byrne and Edmonds, 1990; Shepherd et al., 2010). Often a woman will show signs of her cervix being fully dilated and then just go to sleep, with a contraction every 10 minutes or so. This latent phase is quite normal and allows both the mother and baby to rest before the second stage becomes active (Simkin and Ancheta, 2011).

During labour, the baby descends in the birth canal and the pressure of being squeezed down a tight passage, physically, causes meconium to be passed. This looks very like toothpaste being squeezed out of a tube and is diagnostic of a breech-presenting baby and is a normal anatomical process and is not a sign that the baby is distressed. Any other type of meconium-stained liquor should be considered as with a cephalic birth (Page, 2000). Meconium-stained liquor with other signs of compromise means the plan in place may have to be reconsidered.

Careful monitoring of the baby should start in the antenatal period to learn what the baby's 'normal' heart rate is. Cardiotocography is not recommended for normal labour (NICE, 2014). Intermittent auscultation with a Pinnard stethoscope, a fetascope, a stethoscope or a hand-held Doppler is acceptable to most women. Knowing how the baby is coping with labour helps inform decisions for the birth.

Delivery/birth

> ### Practice points
>
> - Detailed, open counselling assists the parents with their decisions.
> - The baby should be 37–42 weeks gestation when labour starts.
> - Well-grown babies have a similar bi-trochanteric to bi-parietal diameter ratio.
> - A quiet, calm atmosphere is essential for the physiology of labour to progress smoothly.
> - Well-supported women, with an unmedicated labour, will usually adopt a position that aids their anatomy and physiology to progress to a spontaneous birth.
> - Observe the woman's spontaneous movements that aid flexion of the baby.
> - Spontaneous pushing is optimal – avoid the Valsalva manoeuvre.

The standard teaching for a breech delivery is for the woman to be in the lithotomy position and for the baby to be manoeuvred during the delivery, which has the potential to cause damage. It is becoming accepted practice, worldwide, for the woman to adopt an all-fours position for a breech birth, as with a cephalic birth.

An upright position for the second stage of labour has many advantages – there is less risk of cord compression when the baby is in an anterior position, the uterus is in an optimal position for efficient contractions, the woman's sacrum is not compressed against the bed, the woman's pelvis is more mobile and can open fully, the woman can spontaneously move to assist the birth, the birth is aided by gravity with no manoeuvres being required, and the birth occurs spontaneously (Lawrence et al., 2013; Reitter et al., 2014). Many obstetricians experienced with breech birth in an upright position have formed the opinion that breech birth should be the work of the midwife within the context of normality.

When the active second stage has started, most women spontaneously move into an upright, forward-leaning, kneeling position or a squat. These are optimal positions for mobility by using gravity to assist the birth. Some women stand but a small study of standing breech births, begun in the UK in the late 1990s found that early separation of the placenta was more common when the women were standing, which compromised the babies. The study was stopped but was cited in a textbook (Lewis, 2004). The study was very small but many experienced midwives have found their experience supports the findings, and

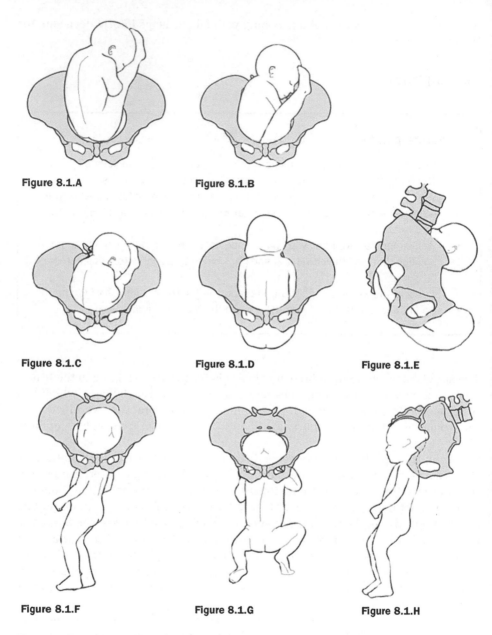

Figure 8.1.A

Figure 8.1.B

Figure 8.1.C

Figure 8.1.D

Figure 8.1.E

Figure 8.1.F

Figure 8.1.G

Figure 8.1.H

Figure 8.1 The normal mechanisms of breech birth.

Source: Jane Evans and Philippa Evans.

early separation of the placenta appears to occur more frequently when women stand, so this position is not advised in the UK. Worldwide, some practitioners support women who choose to birth when standing, with good results (Banks, 1998).

During the second stage, the woman will spontaneously bear down. Directive pushing and use of the Valsalva manoeuvre should be avoided, as this is harmful to both mother and baby (Simkin and Ancheta, 2011).

Women will often spontaneously sit back onto their heels opening the pelvis, flattening the perineal body and flexing the baby into a good position. The mother will not sit on the baby any more than is required to help the baby into an optimal, flexed position, so this movement should not be discouraged.

Once the baby is visible, the birth attendant should take note of the colour of the advancing baby. The anterior buttock is the presenting part when the baby is an extended breech, the most common breech position. The baby will have rotated from the right sacrum anterior (RSA) to the right sacrum lateral/transverse (RSL/T) position (Figure 8.1.B).

With continued descent and lateral flexion of the baby's hips, the genital cleft and the posterior buttock are born. Once the bi-trochanteric diameter (the widest part of the breech) of the baby is past the perineum, 'rumping' has occurred.

The baby then starts to turn from RSL/T to RSA (Figure 8.1.C) and, with continued descent, rotates to direct sacrum anterior (DSA) (Figure 8.1.D). Descent continues with the contractions and the spontaneous, expulsive efforts of the mother. The baby's knees can appear to be bending the wrong way as the baby extends its pelvis round the maternal symphysis pubis (Figure 8.1.E) but the knee caps are very small at this stage of life, so this movement can be accommodated. Inside, this extension movement brings the baby's head and shoulders back a little, past the maternal sacral prominence, while spontaneously releasing the legs and feet from the perineum.

The umbilical cord will now be visible and its vitality, the tone of the baby as it moves, the reperfusion and its colour should be noted. These observations are necessary, as the fetal heart rate cannot be heard abdominally as descent occurs. Neither the cord nor the baby should be touched to avoid stimulation or spasm, which could compromise the baby.

The baby's chest will appear folded, with a cleft, as it is born and this will indicate that the arms, which are not yet visible, are in front of the baby. The cord usually runs up this cleft. Rarely, cord occlusion occurs as the shoulders come into the bony pelvis, so careful observation of the baby is imperative.

The baby continues to descend and rotate from DSA to left sacrum anterior (LSA) (Figure 8.1.F). During this descent and rotation, the anterior arm is released under the maternal symphysis pubis. The second arm follows soon after and the shoulders are born. It is at this point that there is most risk of cord occlusion, as the baby's head descends into the pelvis during the birth of the shoulders.

Now the head is in the pelvis, the baby rotates back to DSA, and a fit healthy baby will make one or more 'tummy tuck' movements by bringing its arms and legs up towards its head and bringing the shoulders forward (Figure 8.1.G). This movement flexes the baby's head, and brings its chin downward, towards its chest. Inside the pelvis, this movement rolls the baby's occiput on the internal aspect of the maternal symphysis pubis and the mother is impelled to drop her torso from upright to horizontal. This movement must be completely spontaneous and brings the mother's pelvis round the baby's head and thus releases the baby from her pelvis and then from her perineum (Evans, 2012a, 2012b) (Figure 8.1.H). If there is no room for her to drop forwards, she will bring her buttocks backward, which has a similar effect.

A physiological third stage is optimal, leaving the cord intact until pulsation has stopped (Mercer et al., 2008; Mercer and Erikson-Owens, 2010; Pilley Edwards and Wickham, 2011). Breech babies will often need a moment or two to recover. Most recover spontaneously, some with the stimulation of drying while some will need resuscitation with inflation breaths. Very occasionally the baby will need further treatment and require admission to neonatal intensive care for a day or two.

An example of a breech birth can be seen by following through Figures 8.2 to 8.13.

HANNAH'S BIRTH

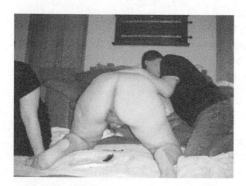

Figure 8.2 Baby 'rumping'.

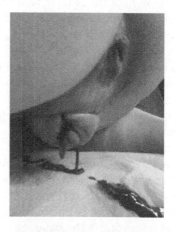

Figure 8.3 Baby 'rumping'.

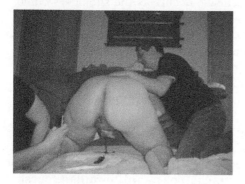

Figure 8.4 Mum rising and dropping to encourage descent of the baby.

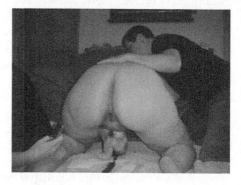

Figure 8.5 Legs being released, mum low down so baby sitting on the floor.

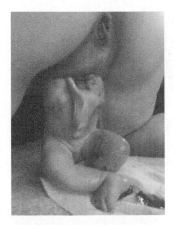

Figure 8.6 Baby sitting on the floor (flexion encouraged).

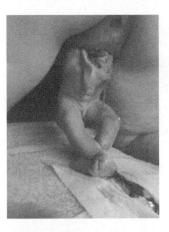

Figure 8.7 Mum has moved up to give baby more space (arm at introitus).

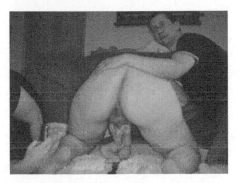

Figure 8.8 Baby still sitting on the floor and flexing with first arm at the intriotus.

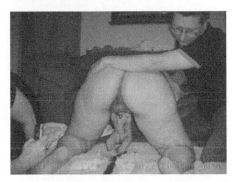

Figure 8.9 Mum has lifted instinctively to give more space.

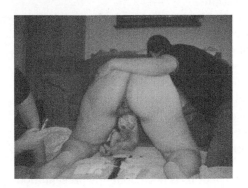

Figure 8.10 Baby doing a 'tummy scrunch' and lifting her arms and legs.

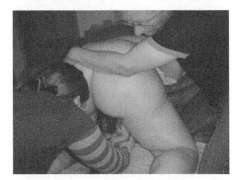

Figure 8.11 Head of the baby born. Baby received by midwife and passed through to mum.

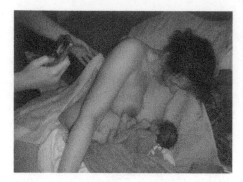

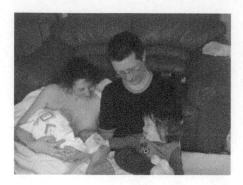

Figure 8.12 First feed – note the legs in the same position as in utero.

Figure 8.13 Happy family.

Source: All images. Jane Evans. With permission from Amy Weatherup.

Non-optimal presentations

With any slightly 'different' presentation, there are signs that will indicate the baby is not in an optimal position. This does not mean that the baby cannot be born spontaneously, but it will require careful observation of maternal and fetal wellbeing and of continued progress and a readiness to help if needed.

The baby in a LSA position will mirror the mechanisms until the rotations to deliver the arms. When the baby is RSA, the rotations bring the arm that was posterior at the start of labour round to become the anterior arm and, therefore, the first to be born. This appears as a natural Lovsett's manoeuvre.

When the baby is LSA, it will usually rotate back from DSA to LSA. This means the arms do not complete the rotation and it is often the posterior arm that is born first, with the anterior arm becoming delayed on the maternal symphysis pubis. It is believed that the internal soft tissues and the bony architecture of the maternal pelvis influence the positioning and the rotations.

Often the baby in LSA and occasionally in RSA just descends through the pelvis and makes no rotations. These babies will often require some help to be born, as the lack of rotations indicates a possible obstruction.

The posterior buttock or genitalia should not be the presenting part, as this will indicate a slight deflexion of the baby. The mechanisms of the birth (described above), the movements of mother and baby, and the rotations of the baby will usually continue, whatever part of the baby presents initially. Some will make a complete rotation of the pelvis, with descent, before being born. Patient, careful observation of progress and the wellbeing of the mother and baby are required before any intervention is made.

A foot presenting usually causes concern, but this is not a common presentation (RCOG, 2006). There is often a misdiagnosis of a 'footling' breech when it is in fact a 'flexed' breech and the leg is folded but the foot presents just before, or simultaneous to, the buttocks or genitalia. A knee presentation is even more rare than a footling but both, once full dilatation has been reached, can be born vaginally quite normally.

If a foot is extended and presents before full dilatation, the woman can be asked to gently touch the baby's foot and then lie on her side, breathing through her contractions until the cervix is fully dilated. The baby will usually retract its foot and keep it warm, inside the vagina, until full dilatation is reached and the baby can be born. This is possible for primigravid as well as multigravid women.

A knee presentation can also progress to a spontaneous vaginal birth. These babies need to descend in a posterior position, as the knee needs to flex forward, under the maternal symphysis pubis, to be born. The baby will then rotate to a lateral position and then continue with the usual rotations and movements to be born. This presentation is more successful for multiparous women, as a posterior position is less optimal for a primigravida.

Practice points

- Patient, careful observation of progress and wellbeing of mother and baby is crucial throughout the birth.
- It is optimal that the anterior part of the baby should present first and the legs should deliver spontaneously.
- Carefully note the reperfusion, colour and tone of the baby.
- The umbilical cord should be vital, not flaccid and empty or overfull.
- The abdomen should not be extended, as this may indicate an extended head.
- Rotations should occur with descent through the pelvis.
- A visible cleft indicates that the arms are in front of the head.
- The maternal perineum should be full when the shoulders are born, indicating that the head is flexed and ready to be born.

Having described the optimal conditions for breech birth, some babies are born successfully when not everything is optimal. The mother and baby work as a dyad and communicate, with positions and movements that bring the baby to a position from which it can be born. It is only when there is concern for the health of the baby or mother that intervention is required.

How to help

Indications for an intervention include delay in the normal progress of the birth and deterioration in the baby's condition.

Labour delay

After spontaneous onset, labour should progress well, without stopping and starting during the first stage. If labour stops, then there should be discussion about the optimal way of delivering the baby, which may be to have a LSCS (Figure 8.14.A). In the developed world, we have access to safe surgery. The labour may stop when the mother's cervix has reached full dilatation, or even when part of the baby is just visible at the introitus but there is no further progress. Again this would indicate that LSCS is the safest way to deliver the baby, with great care being taken to avoid damage to the uterine arteries as the baby is lifted back out of the pelvis. Practitioners who have experience with breech birth find that 20–35% of planned breech births change to a LSCS delivery (personal communication at Sheffield and Oxford Conferences 2014).

If the bi-trochanteric diameter of the baby has passed through the outlet of the maternal pelvis, then the baby should be able to be born vaginally. Unless there is an urgent need to deliver the baby to avoid compromise, the legs should deliver spontaneously. While they are still in the vagina, the mother is able to drop back and down, as described earlier, and help the baby flex so this is a time to be 'hands off the breech', as releasing the legs makes flexion more difficult.

Delay at the shoulders

Delay at the shoulders in a breech birth may occur and this is the equivalent of a shoulder dystocia with a cephalic birth (Figure 8.14.B). When the baby is descending on the left side of the maternal pelvis and no rotations occur, there is a strong possibility that help will be needed to release the anterior arm held up on the symphysis pubis. With the mother in an upright position, it is best to use the baby's shoulder girdle to manoeuvre the baby (Figure 8.14.B1). Using the baby's pelvic girdle would only twist the waist. As with any impaction, a very slight lift will usually dis-impact the arm and then the baby can be rotated so descent and birth follow.

Louwen, an obstetrician in Germany, experienced in all-fours breech birth, describes the manoeuvre as follows: with one hand either side of the baby's chest, like a prayer position with the baby between the hands, turning the baby one hundred and eighty degrees across the maternal symphysis pubis, bringing the anterior arm off the symphysis pubis, behind the baby's head, and then to turn the baby back ninety degrees to bring the arm in front of the baby and thus the arms can be brought down and delivered. He does this before the posterior arm is born, as it is recognized that the situation is unlikely to resolve itself (Louwen, 2012) (Figure 8.14.B3).

Many experienced midwives wait for the posterior arm to be born and then choose to turn the baby the way it is easiest, even if this turns the baby's face anterior, across the maternal symphysis pubis (Figure 8.14.B2). The delayed arm, after resolution of the impaction, will be in front of the baby's face as rotation and descent occur, so risk of the chin being caught on the symphysis pubis is minimal. The baby will often be seen to make the arm and leg movements that flex the head and the baby rotates round the pelvis from DSP to DSA and is born spontaneously.

After the resolution of the shoulders, some babies will need further help to flex their heads. The baby's shoulders will be born and the head should rotate to bring the occiput directly anterior, behind the maternal symphysis pubis. This is the time that occlusion of the cord is most likely to occur, as the head is entering the pelvis, so careful observation of the colour and tone of the baby as well as the vitality of the cord is of essence. Rotation can be assisted if necessary by sliding your fingers or hand in beside the head and manually rotating the head to bring the occiput behind the maternal symphysis pubis.

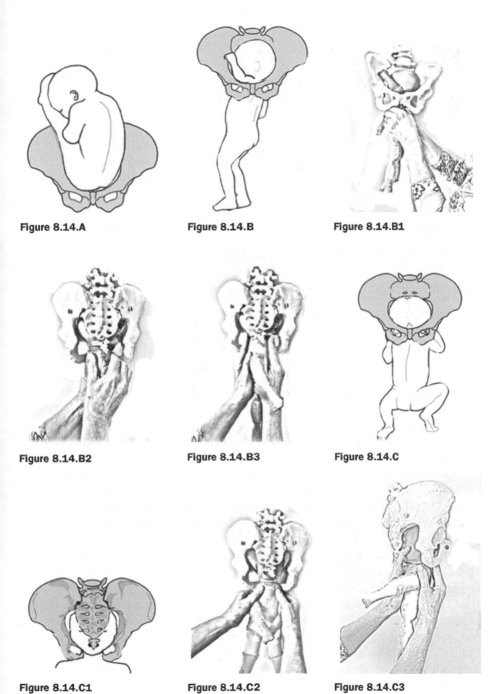

Figure 8.14.A

Figure 8.14.B

Figure 8.14.B1

Figure 8.14.B2

Figure 8.14.B3

Figure 8.14.C

Figure 8.14.C1

Figure 8.14.C2

Figure 8.14.C3

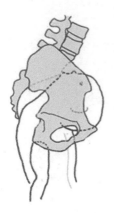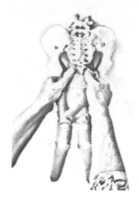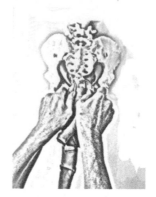

Figure 8.14.D   **Figure 8.14.D1**   **Figure 8.14.D2**

Source: All images in Figure 8.14. Jane Evans and Philippa Evans.

Delay at the head

The baby may have a deflexed head or an extended head that will need help. A deflexed head is when the chin is not on the baby's chest but is in the maternal pelvis (Figures 8.14.C, 8.14.C1). This can occur when the cord is round the neck but is usually easily resolved with either an upward pressure on the occiput or the use of the Mauriceau-Cronk manoeuvre (Frye, 2004), which adds downwards pressure on the cheekbones to flex the head inside the pelvis (Figure 8.14.C3). After flexion has been achieved, with flexion manually maintained, the mother can be asked to drop forwards to bring her pelvis round the baby's head. The baby is then helped to pass the perineum and is passed forwards between the mother's legs where assessment for resuscitation can be made. These babies often recover spontaneously, but they may just need stimulation or need inflation breaths, but it is optimal to perform any resuscitation with the cord intact.

There is an alternative method, described by Louwen (2012) where, once the baby is DSA, pressure is applied to the baby in the sub-clavicular space. This is usually easiest using the thumbs of both hands, with the fingers round the upper arms on the baby's shoulder blades (Figure 8.14.C2). Continuous pressure is then applied, in the sub-clavicular space, pressing the baby towards the maternal symphysis pubis, following the sacral curve, and gradually the head will flex and pass the perineum and be born.

A baby with an extended head will be presenting the same diameter as a brow presentation. The occiput will be held up on the maternal symphysis pubis and the chin wedged against the sacrum or forehead held up on the sacral prominence (Figure 8.14.D). The perineum will be empty and a shadow, from the empty perineum, will be visible on the baby's upper chest. On internal examination, the occiput will be felt, anteriorly, just inside the introitus and the 'bird beak' of the underside of the baby's lower jaw is felt high up in the pelvis, behind the perineum. This position is rare when the labour has been spontaneous.

To resolve this, a similar manoeuvre is used as that for the deflexed head. The baby's head should be moved into a DSA position. The baby should be held with the thumbs in the sub-clavicular space and the hands round the baby's shoulders, with the fingers on the shoulder blades (Figure 8.14.D1). The baby should be minimally lifted to resolve the obstruction/impaction; the thumbs should be pressed into the sub-clavicular space (which releases the sternoclei-domastoid ligament) simultaneously with bringing the shoulders forwards (which releases the cervical vertebrae) to allow the head to flex (Figure 8.14. D2). This manoeuvre can be repeated or held until the face is visible. Once flexion has been achieved, the baby can be delivered in the same way as for a deflexed head, with continued forward pressure round the maternal symphysis pubis – do not pull – or with the Mauriceau-Cronk manoeuvre. These babies do usually need some resuscitation but respond quickly if appropriate action is taken.

If the baby has little tone, supra-pubic pressure may also be applied, by a colleague, after the head has been dis-impacted, with the woman in a kneeling position, to assist the flexion, rotation and descent of the head.

The manoeuvres described in this 'how to help' section of the chapter are rarely required but all professionals should be aware of how to calmly help a breech-presenting baby, if help is required.

Supervision

At the present time, the role of the supervisor in supporting both women and midwives is set out by the NMC (2009). This is clearly demonstrated by the following case study. At the time of writing, however, supervision is under review.

Case 8.2: Lauren

Lauren and Larry were expecting their second child. Having had a quick and easy birth with their first child, they were planning to birth at home with the care of independent midwives. Mid pregnancy the baby was diagnosed as being in a breech position. Lauren accepted a referral to discuss her options at the local unit with an obstetrician and via ultrasound scan it was determined that the baby was in a footling presentation. Lauren was advised to have a LSCS to deliver her baby.

Their midwives also arranged a meeting with a midwife experienced with breech birth and their supervisor. Detailed discussion of their options took place and Lauren and Larry decided they would like to give birth in hospital but did not want a planned LSCS. Unfortunately the hospital declined to support their choice as they advised LSCS. This left Lauren and Larry in the position of having to stay at home with a potentially complicated breech birth or to succumb to a LSCS.

The supervisor of midwives liaised with the local head of midwifery and suggested that the couple would very much like to give birth in hospital, with their midwives, but did not wish to have a LSCS. It was pointed out that it was safer to accommodate Lauren and Larry, as their other option was to remain at home. Honorary contracts were made available to the midwives, and the supervisor also highlighted the fact that the hospital protocols for vaginal breech birth would be inappropriate.

Labour started early one morning and everyone went to the hospital. Lauren was in strong labour and her cervix rapidly progressed to full dilatation; she then started to push. Soon there was a foot visible and then another foot, both with the heel towards Lauren's front. The legs continued to emerge and then the buttocks and the extended abdomen. There was no rotation but there was continuous progress. Lauren then started to drop back onto her heels but this bent the legs back under her as she was on all fours. The experienced midwife managed to flip the legs towards Lauren's back as she started to drop back again. This encouraged the baby to flex and soon there was a movement that was painful for Lauren but she continued to push the baby out. Soon the elbows were visible, then the arms and hands that had been in front of the baby's face and then the baby's head was born and she was passed through to her parents.

No resuscitation was required but it was obvious from the baby's position, which she stayed in for the next few days, that she had been in an extended position and had been 'star-gazing'. The third stage was physiological and the new family went home later the same day.

Without good supervisory support, from a knowledgeable supervisor of midwives and the support of the head of midwifery, this potentially complicated birth would have occurred at home.

Conclusion

To bring breech birth back into normal practice, it is important to develop a supportive network of all professions involved as well as management. A detailed knowledge of the anatomy and physiology and the mechanisms of normal breech birth will help identify when and how to help.

Midwives are the experts in normal childbirth and it is our duty to maintain and regain the ability to safely support women's decisions when they have a breech-presenting baby.

Further reading

Banks, M. (1998) *Breech Birth, Woman Wise*. Hamilton, NZ: Birth Spirit Books. A straightforward, accessible book covering all aspects of breech presentation and breech birth. It is aimed at midwives supporting women who do not want a traditional medicalized approach to their pregnancy, labour and birth that happens to have a breech-presenting baby.

Waites, B. (2003) *Breech Birth*. London: Free Association Books. A book that is useful for parents, midwives and obstetricians. It covers everything related to the experience of breech presentation, including possible causes, turning techniques and options for birth.

References

Banks, M. (1998) *Breech Birth, Woman Wise*. Hamilton, NZ: Birth Spirit Books.

Bogner, G., Strobl, M., Schausberger, C., Fischer, T., Reisenberg er, K. and Jacobs, V.R. (2015) Breech delivery in the all fours position: a prospective observational comparative study with classic assistance, *Journal of Perinatal Medicine*, 43 (6): 707–13.

Borbolla Foster, A., Bagust, A., Bisits, A., Holland, M. and Welsh, A. (2014) Lessons to be learnt in managing the breech presentation at term: an 11-year single-centre retrospective study, *Australian and New Zealand Journal of Obstetrics and Gynaecology*, 54 (4): 333–9.

Byrne, D.L. and Edmonds, D.K. (1990) Clinical method for evaluating progress in first stage of labour, *Lancet*, 335 (8681): 122.

Darmasseelane, K., Hyde, M.J., Santhakumaran, S., Gale, C. and Modi, N. (2014) Mode of delivery and offspring body mass index, overweight and obesity in adult life: a systematic review and meta-analysis, *PLoS One*, 9 (2): e87896.

Evans, J. (2012a) Understanding physiological breech birth, *Essentially MIDIRS*, 3 (2): 17–21.

Evans, J. (2012b) The final piece of the breech birth jigsaw?, *Essentially MIDIRS*, 3 (3): 46–9.

Frye, A. (2004) *Holistic Midwifery: A comprehensive textbook for midwives in homebirth practice, Vol. II: Care from onset of labor through the first hours after birth* (pp. 965–6). Portland, OR: Labrys Press.

Frye, A. (2010) *Healing Passage: A midwife's guide to the care and repair of the tissues involved in birth* (6th edn., pp. 75–93). Portland, OR: Labrys Press.

Garratt, L. (2011) *Survivors of Childhood Sexual Abuse and Midwifery Practice*. Oxford: Radcliffe Publishing.

Glezerman, M. (2006) Five years to the Term Breech Trial: the rise and fall of a randomized controlled trial, *American Journal of Obstetrics and Gynecology*, 194 (1): 20–5.

Goffinet, F., Carayol, M., Foidart, J.M., Alexander, S., Uzan, S., Subtil, D. et al. (2006) Is planned vaginal delivery of breech presentation at term still an option? Results of an observational prospective survey in France and Belgium, *American Journal of Obstetrics and Gynecology*, 194 (4): 1002–11.

Hannah, M.E., Hannah, W.J., Hewson, S.A., Hodnett, E.D., Saigal, S. and Willan, A.R. (2000) Planned caesarean section versus planned vaginal birth for breech presentation at term: a randomised multicentre trial, *Lancet*, 356: 1375–83.

Hannah, M.E., Whyte, H., Hannah, W.J., Hewson, S., Amankwah, K., Cheng, M. et al. (2004) Maternal outcomes at 2 years after planned caesarean section versus planned vaginal birth for breech presentation at term: the International Randomised Term Breech Trial, *American Journal of Obstetrics and Gynecology*, 191 (3): 917–27.

Huang, L., Chen, Q., Zhao, Y., Wang, W., Fang, F. and Bao, Y. (2015) Is elective cesarean section associated with a higher risk of asthma? A meta-analysis, *Journal of Asthma*, 52 (1): 16–25.

Huh, S.Y., Rifas-Shiman, S.L., Zera, C.A., Edwards, J.W., Oken, E., Weiss, S.T. et al. (2012) Delivery by caesarean section and risk of obesity in preschool age children: a prospective cohort study, *Archives of Disabled Children*, 97 (7): 610–16.

Kotaska, A. (2004) Inappropriate use of randomised trials to evaluate complex phenomena: case study of vaginal breech delivery, *British Medical Journal*, 329 (7573): 1039–42.

Larciprete, G., Valensise, H., Di Pierro, G., Vasapollo, B., Casalino, B., Arduini, D. et al. (2005) Intrauterine growth restriction and fetal body composition, *Ultrasound in Obstetrics and Gynecology*, 26 (3): 258–62.

Lawrence, A., Lewis, L., Hofmeyr, G.J. and Styles, C. (2013) Maternal positions and mobility during first stage labour, *Cochrane Database of Systematic Reviews*, 10: CD003934.

Lawson, H.G. (2012) The Term Breech Trial ten years on: primum non nocere?, *Birth*, 39 (1): 3–9.

Lewis, P. (2004) Malpositions and malpresentations, in C. Henderson and S. Macdonald (eds) *Mayes' Midwifery: A textbook for midwives* (13th edn.). Edinburgh: Baillière Tindall.

Louwen, F. (2012) A broader perspective of breech birth, in *Hands 'Off' the Breech: Evidence and practice*, Conference proceedings, 30 November 2012, Sydney, NSW.

Louwen, F., Daviss, B., Johnson, K.C. and Reitter, A. (2016) Does breech delivery in an upright position instead of on the back improve outcomes and avoid cesareans? Available at: http://onlinelibrary.wiley.com/doi/10.1002/ijgo.12033/epdf (accessed 1 December 2016).

Maier, B., Georgoulopoulos, A., Zajc, M., Jaeger, T., Zuchna, C. and Hasenoehrl, G. (2011) Fetal outcome for infants in breech by method of delivery: experiences with a stand-by service system of senior obstetricians and women's choices of mode of delivery, *Journal of Perinatal Medicine*, 39 (4): 385–90.

Mercer, J. and Erikson-Owens, D. (2010) Evidence for neonatal transition and the first hour of life, in D. Walsh and S. Downe (eds) *Essential Midwifery Practice: Intrapartum care*. Chichester: Wiley-Blackwell.

Mercer, J., Skovgaard, R. and Erikson-Owens, D. (2008) Fetal to neonatal transition: first do no harm, in S. Downe (ed.) *Normal Childbirth: Evidence and debate* (2nd edn). Edinburgh: Churchill Livingstone.

National Institute for Clinical Excellence in Health (NICE) (2014) *Intrapartum Care: Care of healthy women and their babies during childbirth*, Clinical Guideline CG190. London: NICE [https://www.nice.org.uk/guidance/cg190].

Nursing and Midwifery Council (NMC) (2009) *Standards for Pre-registration Midwifery*. London: NMC [https://www.nmc.org.uk/standards/additional-standards/standards-for-pre-registration-midwifery-education/].

Nursing and Midwifery Council (NMC) (2012) *Midwives' Rules and Standards*. London: NMC [https://www.nmc.org.uk/standards/additional-standards/midwives-rules-and-standards/].

Odent, M. (2002) *The Farmer and the Obstetrician*. London: Free Association Books.

O'Neill, S.M., Kearney, P.M., Kenny, L.C., Khashan, A.S., Henriksen, T.B., Lutomski, J.E. et al. (2013) Caesarean delivery and subsequent stillbirth or miscarriage: systematic review and meta-analysis, *PLoS One*, 8 (1): e54588.

Page, L.A. (ed.) (2000) *The New Midwifery*. Edinburgh: Churchill Livingstone.

Peel, J. (1970) *Domiciliary Midwifery and Maternity Beds Needs: Report of the Standing Maternity and Midwifery Advisory Committee of the Central Health Services Council*. London. HMSO.

Pilley Edwards, N. and Wickham, S. (2011) *Birthing Your Placenta: The third stage*. Surbiton: AIMS.

Reitter, A., Daviss, B.A., Bisits, A., Schollenberger, A., Vogl, T., Herrmann, E. et al. (2014) Does pregnancy and/or shifting positions create more room in a woman's pelvis?, *American Journal of Obstetrics and Gynecology*, 211 (6): 662: e1–9.

Royal College of Obstetricians and Gynaecologists (RCOG) (2006) *Breech Presentation, Management*, Green-top Guideline No. 20b. London: RCOG [https://www.rcog.org.uk/en/guidelines-research-services/guidelines/gtg20b/; accessed November 2015].

Schutte, J.M., Steegers, E.A., Santema, J.G., Schultemaker, N.W. and van Roosmalen, J. (2007) Maternal deaths after elective cesarean section for breech presentation in the Netherlands, *Acta Obstetrica Gynecologica Scandinavia*, 86 (2): 240–3.

Sevelsted, A., Stokholm, J., Bönnelykke, K. and Bisgaard, H. (2015) Cesarean section and chronic immune disorders, *Pediatrics*, 135 (1): e92–8.

Shepherd, A., Cheyne, H., Kennedy, S., McIntosh, C., Styles, M. and Niven, C. (2010) The purple line as a measure of labour progress: a longitudinal study, *BMC Pregnancy and Childbirth*, 10: 54.

Silver, R.M., Landon, M.B., Rouse, D.J., Leveno, K.J., Spong, C.Y., Thom, E.A. et al. (2006) Maternal morbidity associated with multiple repeat cesarean deliveries, *Obstetrics and Gynecology*, 107 (6): 1226–32.

Simkin, P. and Ancheta, R. (2011) *The Labor Progress Handbook* (3rd edn). Oxford. Wiley-Blackwell.

Turner, M.J. (2006) The Term Breech Trial: are the clinical guidelines justified by the evidence?, *Journal of Obstetrics and Gynaecology*, 26 (6): 491–4.

Whyte, H., Hannah, M., Saigal, S., Hannah, W.J., Hewson, S., Amankwah, K. et al. (2004) Outcomes of children at two years after planned cesarean birth vs. planned vaginal birth for breech presentation at term: the International Randomised Term Breech Trial, *American Journal of Obstetrics and Gynecology*, 191 (3): 864–71.

9

Multiple pregnancy
Kathryn Gutteridge

Introduction

A pregnancy involving more than one fetus is not only a challenge to the woman and her family but also the clinicians providing her care. Although the management of pregnancy in our modern technological society is safer and more evidence-based than ever, the emotional aspect is often neglected or considered secondary to physical care.

This chapter will look at what a multiple pregnancy is usually defined as in the UK and how this is determined. The challenges of a multiple pregnancy will be explored through the woman's perspective but also that of a midwife in modern maternity services. Although a multiple pregnancy can create a number of clinical situations that require intervention, there is still a lot that can be achieved by normalizing care.

Classification of twins and multiples

It is important to know the anatomical features and classification of multiple births, as this will determine antenatal care and also the management of labour and birth. Using ultrasound technology has made it possible to view the developing embryo and all structures that are likely to predict fetal wellbeing. Women and their partners need to understand the typology of their multiple pregnancy and how that might influence their antenatal and intrapartum care.

Often women will disclose a family history of twins during the booking interview, thus alerting the midwife. A degree of anxiety is experienced and is generally normal until visualization of the pregnancy by ultrasonography. The use of ultrasound in any pregnancy is an unquantifiable experience and it is vital that the sonographer engages with the couple throughout the procedure to gauge their understanding and feelings (Mitchell, 2004).

There are some basic facts that can be helpful in understanding twin and multiple births. Before we consider the prevalence of multiple births, some facts about twins will be outlined.

Types of twins

Zygosity is the degree of genetic material contained within the zygote. There are five combinations of twins in terms of zygosity:

Dizygotic

- Male–female twins are most common, representing 50% of all dizygotic twins.
- Female–female dizygotic twins (sometimes called 'sororal twins').
- Male–male dizygotic twins.

Monozygotic

- Female–female monozygotic twins.
- Male–male monozygotic twins (less common).

Dizygotic, binovular or fraternal twins are the most common type of twin births, with around two-thirds of all twins falling into this group. These arise from separate ova fertilized by different spermatozoa and contain differing genetic and DNA information. These pregnancies will usually have two chorions and amnions and two placentae that may be fused; there is no merging of fetal circulation. In around half of cases, the embryos will be of the same sex. In the case of a previous history of twin pregnancies, family genetics and heredity factors will be to the fore (Chiayat and Hall, 2006). Other factors such as age, parity, race, maternal height and weight will also affect the likelihood of such pregnancies (Bortolus et al., 1999). Maternal genetic predisposition is a feature of dizygotic twins, with a predominant family history of ovarian hyperstimulation (Fauser et al., 2005). The twins will have no more chance of sharing the same genetic profile than singleton siblings do; they may have similar features and traits but this is usually because they are the same age and share experiences.

Interestingly, the rate of dizygotic twin pregnancies varies throughout the modern world. Epidemiological studies show that twinning ranges from about 6 per 1000 births in East Asia and Oceania to 15 or more per 1000 in some parts of India, with over 20 per 1000 in some Central African countries (Smits and Monden, 2011). Where higher rates of twinning have been reported, further scrutiny suggests that nutrition, maternal height and the previous number of pregnancies all influence twinning (Oleszczuk et al., 1999).

Monozygotic, uniovular or identical twins are less common than dizygotic, binovular or fraternal twins, with only one-third of twin pregnancies being accounted for by this group. This type of twin pregnancy arises from a single ovum being fertilized by a single spermatozoon; the classification of this group of twins is then further determined by the timing of the split of the zygote. Why the zygote should split is largely unknown but it is apparent that the later it splits, the more complex and likely it is that there is some form of conjoining.

Early splitting of the zygote results in each of the twins having its own amnion, chorion and placenta; these twins are classified as *dichorionic-diamniotic*. Splitting of the zygote at between 4 and 8 days will determine that the twins share placentae and chorionic sac but exist in their own amniotic sac; these are *monochorionic-diamniotic* twins. And splitting of the zygote at between 8 and 12 days will result in shared placentae, chorionic and amniotic sac; these twins are classified as *monoamniotic-monochorionic*.

Most monochorionic pregnancies will have blood vessels that link the placentae, and as long as blood flow is uninhibited, no problem should arise. However, if there are anastamoses between an artery and a vein and blood flow is directed one way only, then *twin-to-twin transfusion* is the outcome (Fisk, 1995). Such transfusion affects approximately 15% of monchorionic-diamniotic twins and results in fetal compromise and stillbirth in 20% of cases (NICE, 2011).

Prevalence of multiple births in the UK

Multiple pregnancies in the UK are quite common, with twin pregnancies forming the majority of these (1 in 80 conceived pregnancies). Triplet pregnancies account for 1 in 6400 births and quadruplets 1 in 700,000 pregnancies, according to Hellin's Law (Fellman and Eriksson, 2009).

In England and Wales, the multiple birth rate was 10,783 in 2013 compared with 12,675 in 2012, a fall in this category of pregnancies (ONS, 2013). However, over the last two decades there has been a consistent rise in the incidence of multiple births; this rise in multiple births has been attributed to the increasingly successful *in vitro* fertilization (IVF) techniques made available to couples (Ozturk and Templeton, 2002; NICE, 2011). Overall in England and Wales, twin and triplet pregnancies constitute approximately 3% of all pregnancies. Although assisted pregnancy techniques are responsible for approximately 24% of pregnancies, natural conception of twin births accounts for 1 in 89 pregnancies (Fellman and Eriksson, 2009).

The incidence of multiple pregnancies following IVF techniques has fallen based on recommendations in the Human Fertilization and Embryology Act 2008 that the number of embryos transferred to women undergoing *in vitro* fertilization be reduced from three to two. While assisted fertility does affect the number of multiple births, the incidence of natural multiple conception increases with some maternal factors (Beemsterboer et al., 2006).

There is a natural prevalence of multiple conceptions in women aged 35–39 years; one theory for this is that older women produce a higher level of follicle stimulating hormone, or FSH (Utting and Bewley, 2011). The ovaries are slower to respond to FSH, thus multiple ova are produced, causing multiple follicular development. In the presence of two good quality oocytes, a twin pregnancy is likely (Beemsterboer et al., 2006).

Technology confirming multiple pregnancies

Today, women take for granted the use of technology in their pregnancies; in fact, it could be said they expect it (NICE, 2014). When a multiple pregnancy is suspected, screening and ultrasonography are the standard to determine all relevant features.

NICE guidance advocates first trimester ultrasound to determine gestational age, the optimum timing being between 11 weeks and 13 weeks + 6 days (NICE, 2011). The aim is to identify gestational age, determine chorionicity and to screen for markers of Down's syndrome. Ultrasonography will also define the nomenclature or which twin is sited on the upper or lower region of the uterus; this will be assigned at each ultrasound assessment for consistency.

Determining the 'T-sign' and the 'lambda' is part of early surveillance requirements for managing twin pregnancies. Identification of a 'T-sign' at the inter-twin membrane–placental junction is indicative of monochorionic-diamniotic twins, whereas dichorionic twins present with a 'lambda (λ) sign' where the chorion forms a wedge-shaped protrusion into the inter-twin space, creating a rather curved junction. Where there is indistinct chorionicity and a second opinion cannot provide confirmation, the pregnancy must be determined as monochorionic until proved otherwise (NICE, 2011).

Once initial ultrasonography has determined chorionicity, the pregnancy is to be managed according to the best available evidence and within a care network. Patterns of antenatal care for twin pregnancies are guided by fetal medicine and ultrasonography; while this development in obstetrics has advanced successful multiple births, there is an emotional context that women describe (Breathnach et al., 2011).

Usually, multiple pregnancies are referred to fetal medicine services or multiple clinics, thus ensuring that clinicians working in these services are familiar with the nuances and needs of the women requiring care. A midwife working alongside a fetal medicine obstetrician is a vital asset; this is where the woman's pregnancy is influenced by midwifery advice and support.

There will be instances where a woman declines routine screening and also advice in respect of early induction. It is important that clinicians listen and understand the woman's perspective, ensuring she has all of the relevant information to make her own decisions regarding care of herself and her pregnancy. Sometimes clinicians highlight threats to the fetuses and even fetal demise, but the use of coercion or even manipulation is unhelpful and will result in the sullying of a good patient–clinician relationship (Devaseelan and Ong, 2010; Dagustu, 2012).

Physical changes in multiple-birth pregnancy

A woman with a multiple pregnancy will have many questions about her changing body. There may be early signs that suggest that the pregnancy is not without problems; these include excessive nausea and vomiting, excessive tiredness, weight gain, increasing fundal growth and disproportionate fetal movements.

Minor disorders associated with early pregnancy may be more extreme due to higher levels of human chorionic gonadotropin (hCG) compared with singleton pregnancies. This is an unreliable diagnostic tool, however, and usually directs the clinician to use other screening methods to confirm a multiple pregnancy (Chung et al., 2006).

136 KATHRYN GUTTERIDGE

The size of the uterus is almost the same as in a singleton pregnancy until the second trimester; after week 18, it is twice the size of a singleton pregnancy and, by week 25, the same size as a term singleton pregnancy. This gives some idea of the rapid changes and adjustments that a woman's body has to make. Furthermore, the volume of amniotic fluid is greater in multiple than in singleton pregnancies; it increases markedly until the second trimester and then stabilizes during the beginning of the third trimester, decreasing between weeks 33 and 36.

It is important for women with a multiple pregnancy to have information about nutrition and lifestyle management so that optimum health is maintained. It is recommended that women follow a normal healthy diet and take the normal nutritional supplements as and when recommended (Ballard et al., 2011). Physiological changes in multiple pregnancy are shown in Table 9.1.

Practice point

Knowledge about the physiological changes in women's bodies experiencing multiple pregnancy is important in midwifery. Continuing to offer guidance and support is crucial, and will enable women to have more control over their pregnancy. A simple explanation of why her body is affected in this way can make all the difference, not only for the woman's psychical health but also her emotional wellbeing.

Emotional context of multiple-birth pregnancy

Although pregnancy is associated with psychological adjustment and lability of mood, the degree of change is difficult to quantify. The shock of confirming a multiple pregnancy has the potential to cause high levels of stress for the woman as she enters a pathway of care that is determined as 'high risk' and becomes engaged in an obstetrically driven programme of screening. Attributing a pregnancy as 'high risk' begins a subtle process of destabilizing the woman's belief systems in her own ability to cope with pregnancy, birth her babies and ultimately feed and care for them (Elbourne et al., 1989; Eganhouse and Petersen, 1998; Dagustu, 2012). In the case of a woman handing control over to clinicians, the potential for psychological powerlessness is increased, creating a dependency for reassurance and support (Williams, 2011).

Pregnancy is accepted as a time of major psychological transition and there are documented historical accounts that all women, irrespective of their pregnancy label, experience some degree of anxiety, worry and even fear (Newton, 1955). The neurochemical and biological changes that occur naturally are necessary to generate a sense of 'safe passage' through pregnancy and birth (Rubin, 1975). However, modern midwifery theorists dispute this supposition by stating it is too simplistic, arguing that fetal dominance has the potential to overwhelm and reduce the woman's psychological needs, making them secondary to those of her unborn baby (Parratt and Fahy, 2011).

Table 9.1 Physiological changes in multiple pregnancy.

Physical changes	Rationale	Midwifery explanation	Advice/support
Circulatory changes	Increase in circulatory volume > 35% above singleton pregnancy.	Ensure woman understands the reason she may be experiencing some of the signs and symptoms.	Get up from a lying position slowly, especially after sleep.
	Blood flow through the pregnant uterus increases 20- to 40-fold compared with singleton pregnancy.		Take regular rest periods during the day.
	Decrease in diastolic blood pressure due to increased progesterone causing decreased vascular resistance and increased prevalence of postural hypotension.	Postural hypotension can be unpredictable and cause women to feel afraid and nervous about being away from home.	If feet are swollen, ensure that feet are higher than hips to encourage venous return.
		Varicose veins might look unsightly and cause aching legs.	If varicose veins are painful or inflamed, advise to seek treatment from GP.
	Increased heart rate.	Haemorrhoids can be painful and cause constipation. Prolapsed haemorrhoids may cause bleeding during bowel movements.	Advise a high-fibre diet and increase fluid intake of water. Advise topical treatment that may be used to reduce soreness – however, GP treatment may be required.
	Lower limbs have decreased vasculature resistance and venous return – varicose veins, haemorrhoids and vulval varicosities.		
	Increased nasal congestion and nosebleeds.		
Respiratory changes	Total lung capacity, residual volume and expiratory reserve volume are all decreased, respiratory rate and mean inspiratory flow are unchanged.	Increased capacity in the lungs ensures that women are able to supply the placenta with optimum levels of oxygen for the twins to develop and grow.	Conversation about how the lungs increase in size will help.

(continued)

Table 9.1 (*Continued*).

Physical changes	Rationale	Midwifery explanation	Advice/support
	The increase of ventilation during pregnancy results from hormonal changes and increased carbon dioxide production (which is sensitive to progesterone). Ventilator drive is increased during pregnancy (due to the direct stimulatory effect of progesterone).	Some women experience breathlessness, which may be due to the rapid growth of the fetuses during the second and third trimesters. This is especially uncomfortable for women who are shorter and have a smaller frame.	If breathlessness occurs during exercise, advise moderation and small changes to the way it is taken. For example, walk down stairs only and take the lift up stairs. If breathless during rest, a medical review is required.
Gastrointestinal changes	Increase in salivation and production of saliva. Frequency of gastric emptying is increased in multiple pregnancy. Displacement of the stomach due to the uterus increases gastric return and heartburn symptoms.	Heartburn and other reflux problems can cause distress, particularly when sickness occurs. Women often self-treat by buying treatments from pharmacies or supermarkets.	Explain to women the reasons behind this body change. Advise small but frequent meals. Avoid high fat content in food. Eat larger meals early in the day rather than late at night. Eat bland food if nausea and sickness continue to be an issue. If certain foods increase the reflux, avoid in future

Table 9.1 *(Continued).*

Physical changes	Rationale	Midwifery explanation	Advice/support
Renal changes	Glomerular filtration rate (GFR) increases by approximately 50% by the end of the first trimester to a peak of around 180 mL/min. There are no other renal differences between singleton and multiple pregnancies unless there is underlying maternal renal disease.	Increased urine output is noted quite early in the first trimester of pregnancy and also again at the end of pregnancy. This can cause tiredness and frustration when sleep is interrupted. Occasionally, some women will experience incontinence due to multiparity and multiple pregnancy.	Advise how the bladder and uterus are closely situated and space is optimized. Advise to empty bladder before going to bed even in urge is not felt. Advise that afternoon rest can help with disturbed night sleep. If incontinence is an issue, advise wearing liners to avoid embarrassment. Refer to incontinence service for support and management.
Haematological changes	Increase of approximately 30% of red blood cell mass to compensate for increases in circulatory volume and dilutional effect. Number of erythrocytes increases approximately 25% versus a singleton pregnancy. Due to dilution, platelet levels decrease. Anaemia is more likely in multiple pregnancies.	Increased demand upon red blood cells can show as marked anaemic changes early in multiple pregnancies. This may be exacerbated by previous anaemia, which has not been managed through diet alone.	The woman should understand that if she is anaemic, she will feel increasingly tired and even breathless with a rapid pulse. Diet and nutrition advice is invaluable, particularly if a vegetarian. May require iron replacement treatment; midwifery management of regular blood testing of haemoglobin and other iron studies is important to ensure absorption.

(continued)

Table 9.1 (Continued).

Physical changes	Rationale	Midwifery explanation	Advice/support
Breast changes	Proliferation of milk glands and ducts. Nipples enlarge, areolar pigmentation and development of tubules of Montgomery. Leakage of fluid from nipples. Tenderness and sensitivity to touch.	Early breast changes are one of the first signs of a pregnancy. Women more often than not are aware very quickly of this change. Production of colostrum pre-birth can be disturbing. Milk gland development might cause some women concern, particularly if they feel lumpy.	Explain that breast development is vital for the preparation of infant feeding. Pre-birth leakage is normal and should be explained as a reassuring factor for breastfeeding. Some medical conditions will require birth to be induced early; in these situations, breast milk may be collected early to store for after the birth. Women should meet with the infant feeding team to prepare for this. Reassure women that breasts will produce enough milk for more than one baby and that it is not size-dependent.
Skin changes	Pigmentation, especially of midline of abdomen. Striae is markedly greater than in a singleton pregnancy due to rapid uterine growth. Early signs of ankle and finger oedema.	Body embarrassment is not unusual in pregnancy but the potential is greater in multiple pregnancies. The increased stretch of the uterus and therefore the abdomen will cause more striae. This is also the case for breasts and thighs.	Explain that this process is due to hormone changes and not just fat deposits. Advise that once pregnancy is over, stretch marks will reduce and become less visible over time. Advise women to talk about their concerns and worries.

Table 9.1 (Continued).

Physical changes	Rationale	Midwifery explanation	Advice/support
Musculoskeletal changes	Laxity of ligaments. Pelvic girdle pain increased and presents earlier in multiple pregnancy due to uterine weight and number of fetuses.	Increased laxity is common during multiple pregnancies and often felt earlier during the pregnancy. Common areas that cause pain and discomfort are the suprapubic and sacroiliac regions.	Advise women about support wear that can help. Advise women about positions of comfort when lying and walking. Refer to obstetric physiotherapist if available and symptoms are continuing. May require multidisciplinary team support if severe and unremitting pain.

Source: Gutteridge (2013).

Parenting and multiple babies

Once a multiple pregnancy is confirmed, it is not unusual for a woman to be over-whelmed with fear and anxiety as to how she will perform as a mother and cope, which may be further exacerbated if there are other children in the family. A multiple pregnancy, therefore, has the potential to destabilize relationships within the family. Bonding and attachment, which generally start in pregnancy, are more complex with multiple births; one fetus may not be developing as well as the other, and it is possible that the woman will detach herself emotionally even during pregnancy – a self-protecting phenomenon (Raphael-Leff, 2005). The forming of attachments to mono-zygotic twins is further complicated when babies look identical; parents may assume that the two infants have the same personality and preferences. Dressing and feeding infants the same are a common behaviour but midwives should advise that this could lead to a conflict of identities; wearing bracelets to ensure each child is identifiable is an easy solution to developing individual identities.

Encouraging parents to observe closely individual behaviours is one way midwives can influence equal parenting. Displaying favouritism to one baby is important to note during postnatal care; this often happens if one baby was stron-ger or more robust at birth. In contrast, a baby may have required some neonatal support at birth and therefore the mother may pamper that baby more; this uncon-scious behaviour naturally ensures that the weaker sibling is handled more and the threshold for being ignored is less.

Theories around the complexity of women favouring one baby over another have been around for many years. John Bowlby, one of the major influences on attachment theory, talks about 'monotropy' – a favoured or innate relationship with one child (Bowlby, 1988). Midwives and neonatal staff should be alert to the way parents care for their newborn babies and observe if there is a preference for one of the babies. Babies should be kept together at all times when practical and should go home together. In the case of one twin being discharged earlier than the other, studies have shown maternal preference has focused on that twin to the detriment of the other (Klaus et al., 1995).

Managing emotions, expectations and grief

It is evident that emotions have a greater potential for ebb and flux with a multiple pregnancy. Just the screening journey alone is often more intense and that is with-out the complications that some women experience when one fetus has an identi-fied problem. The fantasies and expectations of women are predetermined to some extent prior to becoming pregnant, throughout their childhood and adoles-cence (Raphael-Leff, 2005). However, these desires and unconscious expectations are escalated in the first few weeks of pregnancy and moderated by fear and dreams of being out of control.

Thorpe et al. (1991) warns that women experiencing twin pregnancies are almost 1.8 times more likely to develop depression during the twins' early years. In the case of triplets, this risk increases five-fold and where there are bereave-ment issues due to fetal loss, the risk increases yet again.

Anomalies and developing fetal problems are increased in multiple pregnancies, hence the reliance upon early and continued fetal screening using sonography. As twins are more common in women over the age of 35 and women seeking fertility treatment, the incidence of chromosomal problems increases in dizygotic twins in particular. Whereas the risk of fetal anomaly in the dizygotic group is the same as with a singleton pregnancy, it increases four-fold in the case of monozygotic pregnancies (Harper et al., 2013). Subsequently, women with multiple pregnancies may have to face invasive tests such as amniocentesis, fetal reduction and the premature death of one or more fetuses.

The woman and her partner may experience a multitude of emotions as they navigate screening systems, consider tests results and try to decide what they should do next. Where hard choices have to be made about pregnancies with fetal anomalies or life-threatening conditions, the woman and her partner need support and access to high-quality psychological care (Devalseelan and Ong, 2010). Women who are identified as having twin-to-twin syndrome will often be referred to tertiary centres where a range of procedures may be discussed and offered to them. At this point, it is possible for a woman to lose contact with all of her local clinicians, especially the midwife, although the midwife may contact the unit and get updates from the new team. Arranging to see the woman in her own home at a convenient time to catch up is another way of maintaining some normality and local support.

Best evidence suggests that intrauterine death and stillbirth in multiple pregnancies are 2–5 times higher than in singleton pregnancies (Skeie et al., 2003; NICE, 2011). Furthermore, stillbirth and neonatal death rates are significantly higher in monochorionic twins than in dichorionic twins (44.2 vs. 12.2 per thousand births in a study of twin and multiple pregnancies in the North of England; Ward Platt et al., 2006). NICE guidance acknowledges that overall the stillbirth rate in multiple pregnancies is higher than in singleton pregnancies: in 2009 the stillbirth rate was 12.3 per thousand twin births and 31.1 per thousand triplet and higher-order multiple births, compared with 5 per thousand singleton births (NICE, 2011).

Elective delivery can also be a difficult thing to discuss, particularly where the woman has prepared herself for an end date to her pregnancy. Schneuber et al. (2011) found that the phenomenon of the second twin was a concept used to discuss bringing forward elective delivery times and has the potential to create anxiety both among clinicians and the women. Careful discussion with a neonatologist, obstetrician and midwife is important where delivery may compromise the wellbeing of the baby after birth. Midwifery involvement here is very important, as the midwife can help the woman prepare, by providing information on breast milk harvesting, for example (East et al., 2014).

Value of midwifery support

The support of a midwife at this time offers many advantages, if only to assist in complex explanations or to help navigate the complex system of maternity screening (Carrick-Sen et al., 2014). Women may have multiple hospital appointments where they meet different clinicians; although this may be important in the scheme of providing appropriate antenatal care, getting to know a community midwife who will listen, support and guide the woman through her pregnancy has endless benefits (Ekström et al., 2015).

There is a greater tendency for anxiety and stress-based disorders in multiple pregnancies, which may lead to a number of psychological and psychiatric states. The quality standards for care published by NICE (2013) stress the need to support and emotionally sustain couples who are experiencing a multiple pregnancy and for them to have access to a specialist midwife.

There is a risk in multiple pregnancy that as a result of less contact with midwives, women are less exposed to the normal antenatal education and routine support generally offered during pregnancy. It is vital that midwives maintain contact with women who have a confirmed multiple pregnancy so that a focus on woman-centred care is maintained. Although NICE recommend that care is delivered by a multidisciplinary team, that team can consist of at least six clinicians; another recommendation is that hospital visits are kept to a minimum and that contact is made near to the woman's home.

Another useful resource for couples experiencing multiple pregnancies is to point them in the direction of support and education advice. There are many organizations that produce literature and booklets for parents but also support groups – both virtual and real. The midwife should be directing prospective parents to look at these early in their pregnancy to provide ideas of how they will manage the challenges along the way (a list of these is presented at the end of the chapter).

Practice point

It is important that women who have uncomplicated twin pregnancies are cared for as near to home as possible and that they are cared for by a team that includes a midwife. This ensures that a relationship of trust can be developed and the benefits of midwifery antenatal care experienced.

The multidisciplinary team

One of the quality standards for multiple pregnancies is the team of clinicians designated to care for women. NICE Quality Standard #46 (2013) indicates that they must include at least:

- a specialist obstetrician who works regularly with women experiencing twin and triplet pregnancies;
- a specialist midwife who has a specialist interest and expertise in supporting women with multiple pregnancies; and
- an ultrasonographer who is skilled at interpreting obstetric ultrasound.

In addition to the above, tertiary units will have access to fetal medicine specialist obstetric services that may be necessary if the chorionicity is determined as more complex in aetiology. Fetal medicine services will also be necessary where amniocentesis, intrauterine interventions and feticide are planned.

Most multiple-birth pregnancies will deliver in units that have access to a neonatal service staffed by a range of neonatal clinicians. During the pregnancy, the team may become involved early because premature labour is more likely or if any of the aforementioned procedures are planned.

Enhanced services suggested by NICE (2011) include a dietician for nutritional advice, perinatal mental health services, an infant feeding advisor and access to an obstetric physiotherapist.

Aims of the multidisciplinary team

- Early contact to maximize care during pregnancy.
- Access to screening and diagnostics to identify gestation, determine chorionicity and screen for anomalies such as Down's syndrome.
- Agree and explain a pathway of care the woman can expect.
- Minimize the number of hospital visits and ensure continuity of care.

Suggested antenatal contact visits

The number of visits a woman will receive during her pregnancy will depend on the type of multiple pregnancy and any complications that may arise. However, NICE (2011) suggest the following:

- women with uncomplicated monochorionic-diamniotic twin pregnancies have at least nine antenatal appointments;
- women with uncomplicated dichorionic twin pregnancies have at least eight antenatal appointments;
- women with uncomplicated monochorionic-triamniotic and dichorionic-triamniotic triplet pregnancies have at least 11 antenatal appointments;
- women with uncomplicated trichorionic-triamniotic triplet pregnancies have at least seven antenatal appointments; and
- women with a twin or triplet pregnancy involving a shared amnion should be offered individualized care by a consultant in a tertiary-level fetal medicine centre.

During these appointments, ultrasonography is performed to assess fetal growth parameters and a full antenatal check undertaken. It is important that the feelings and needs of the woman are not overlooked; it is easy to focus all of the appointments on fetal wellbeing, whereas from a midwifery perspective, the woman should be the first priority.

It is easy to see how women with multiple pregnancies are divorced from their community midwife after the initial booking history appointment, but this is exactly why midwifery contact should be maintained. The normal antenatal input from community midwives will ensure that women with multiple pregnancies have access to advice and support from a range of routine services. This might be antenatal education and meeting other couples where the woman is pregnant, as the sharing of experiences is vital in maintaining a sense of normality when going through new life events (Ekström et al., 2015). The community midwife will also provide postnatal care and therefore contact and continuity of care are important.

Intrapartum care and birth

During the antenatal period and as part of the regular appointment schedule with the multidsicplinary team, discussions will have taken place about the signs of premature labour and what that might entail. A plan must be agreed with the woman about the optimum timing and place for her to give birth and what that may mean for her care during labour. It is generally accepted that if there is more than one fetus *in utero*, labour may begin earlier. This likely means encountering the problems associated with premature labour and need for transfer to a tertiary unit.

Management of labour

Although multiple pregnancies will present many challenges for the clinicians involved in intrapartum care, the priority for these women will be no different to women with a singleton pregnancy. As is generally the case, where doctors and midwives are involved in team working, a balance has to be achieved with the woman about her needs and aspirations for the birth.

One of the most common debates centres on the timing of a twin birth and whether to induce labour or advocate pre-labour caesarean section (Dodd et al., 2010). Breathnach et al. (2010) provide key criteria for conservative labour management that include: vertex-vertex presentation, maternal age, multiparity, and natural conception. These characteristics are known to influence spontaneous labour and good maternal/fetal outcomes. Midwives should understand the positive indicators that will suggest a normal birth outcome and help the woman to identify ways of normalizing her labour by focusing on non-pharmacological coping methods and adapting upright positions for the birth.

In terms of delivery time interval, there are expectations that a time limit will be applied; however, Gourheux et al. (2007) argue that this increases the anxiety of both mother and clinicians. Indeed, the uncertainty that exists about the value of elective birth interventions in multiple pregnancies has yet to be addressed (NICE, 2011).

Midwifery is principally a profession where the woman is the priority, and how that woman is supported and represented is vital in developing any care plan. Advocacy is at the heart of good midwifery and this should underpin any plans the woman has for her pregnancy and birth. Caillagh (2014: 9) states: 'the role of the midwife with a multiple pregnancy is fundamentally no different than that with a singleton'. She also highlights that a midwife caring for a woman with a multiple pregnancy should ask themselves some basic questions about knowledge and skills.

Reflection points

- How skilled am I in examining the landscape of the pregnant uterus with multiple fetuses?
- How much anatomical knowledge do I have regarding this type of pregnancy?
- Do I fully understand the different possible combinations of twins/triplets/ multiples?
- Am I able to detect any abnormal features that the pregnancy is showing?
- Do I understand the physiological adjustments as the pregnancy nears term?
- What do I know about the contracting uterus of a multiple pregnancy?

The above are a few soul-searching questions that a midwife might consider when undertaking care of a multiple pregnancy birth. The following case is an example of a woman expecting a monozygotic twin pregnancy in a midwife-led setting.

Case 7.1: Alexandra

Alexandra was a 41-year-old G2P1 British woman who had her first child abroad 3 years before her twin pregnancy. A monozygotic pregnancy was confirmed by ultrasound early on (12 weeks) and subsequent scans showed fetal anatomy of both twins normal with consistent growth.

Alexandra was keen to have a midwife-led birth in a midwife-only facility (a birth centre). She visited five separate maternity units until she found somewhere nearby when she was 32 weeks pregnant. Under current UK maternity provision, clinicians have become risk-focused and operate in a framework of defensive practice. Exposure to women who have very clear ideas about what they want for their care causes some clinicians concern; their response to such requests is often to adopt coercive language (Dagustu, 2012). Despite this, women continue to seek care with services or midwives who are willing to listen to them and provide supportive care.

The birth

At around 36 weeks gestation, Alexandra knew that her body was starting to labour; she had experienced a restless night and was beginning to feel some tightening and discomfort in her back. Wisely, she kept herself busy – and with a 3-year-old son that was not difficult. By mid-afternoon, Alexandra was sure that today she would start to labour and so she felt she ought alert the birth centre that she may come in.

At 20.00 hours, Alexandra, her husband and their 3-year-old son arrived at the birth centre with positive signs of labour. It was planned that two midwives and a maternity support worker would support the family in their labour and also that the consultant midwife and supervisor of midwives would be informed. Alexandra had clarified all of her birth wishes prior to labour and therefore she made herself comfortable in her birthing room (with her small son tucked up in a travel cot in the corner of the room). The lights were dimmed and Alexandra was very quiet and meditated throughout her labour, so it was very difficult to determine if she was indeed in active labour (Walsh and Gutteridge, 2011). This is where the skills in observing labouring women come into play – using skin colour, breathing changes, movements and positions, it is possible to determine positive signs of labour (Gutteridge, 2013).

After about 2 hours in the quiet, dimmed room, Alexandra showed signs of transition, she stood upright and arched her back – known as the 'fetal ejection reflex', first cited by Newton and described by Lemay when observing labouring women (Newton et al., 1966; Lemay, 2005). This change in behaviour and position is significant; unconsciously, women who labour naturally and uninhibited follow those urges and by making this body adjustment can enlarge the pelvis ready for the descent into the birth canal. Kitzinger (2000) describes this among West Indian women, who call the movement 'opening the back' for the same purposes.

A short time later, Alexandra became alert and focused, and announced quietly that she was ready to push her first baby out. She squatted in front of a deep mat and beanbag, and very quickly following her body's natural urges she progressed her pushing to give birth to her first baby girl. Alexandra caught her own baby and took her to her breast straight away. The midwives were very quiet and stayed in a supportive position around her, putting a warm blanket over her shoulders so that she did not produce too much adrenaline and cool quickly. Alexandra stooped to a sitting position and became absorbed in her new baby who had cried after about one minute of birth, her cord still intact and pulsating in line with both parents' wishes.

After approximately 15 minutes, Alexandra became restless and looked uncomfortable and she asked her partner to take the baby in his arms as she felt the second baby would not be long in coming. Alexandra rose to her knees and leant forward on to the beanbag so that her back and perineum were visible in an all-fours position. Within seconds, a bulging bag of membranes could be seen at the introitus and the vertex of the second twin behind those membranes. The consultant midwife was now sitting watching the labour and gave non-verbal signs for everyone to wait and not intervene yet. The membranes disappeared from the introitus and then Alexandra was feeling the urgent need to push, which she did quite gently. Her second baby girl was born with one push and again into her mother's arms.

The birth of the second twin is known to be a challenge and it is also expected that the twin will be lethargic and somewhat surprised to be born

(Gourheux et al., 2007; Scheunber et al., 2011); this is largely due to the rapid descent through the birth canal and subsequent birth. The two twins were in the arms of their mother, close to one another; the second twin seemed to sense the older baby's presence, opening her eyes and in a skin-to-skin hold started to recover.

The passage of the third stage was relatively quiet and nondescript, with Alexandra announcing that she would like to move a little to allow the placenta to be born. The placentae were fused and in fact estimated blood loss was approximately 300 mL, which surprised everyone in the room. Both babies were eventually weighted and separated from their mother and cords, and their weights recorded respectively as 2.65 and 2.52 kg. The two babies breastfed simultaneously, although Alexandra had met antenatally with the infant feeding midwife and had harvested milk to use if required in the early days. After 6 hours of rest, midwifery checks and essential paperwork, babies, mother, partner and 3-year-old were on their way home in need of rest and recuperation.

Everyone involved in Alexandra's care met up later that day to reflect and discuss the births and what we all felt we had learnt from the experience. Some of those thoughts and reflections included:

- It was amazing; she knew what to do even if I didn't! (midwife 1)
- The most difficult bit was the time between twin 1 and 2; I was watching the clock. (midwife 2)
- The membranes bulging and seeing the vertex with the cervix around it was fantastic. I know if I had been anywhere else, I would have ruptured them – who knows what would have happened. (midwife 3)
- I don't think I will see anything like that again – it was awesome. (student midwife)

Case 9.2: Sarah

Sarah was a 34-year-old G4P3 woman who had had all of her previous three births at home under the care of a midwife. Never previously having experienced any complications, Sarah was quite surprised to find her pregnancy this time was demanding and interventionist. Once the aetiology of the twins was identified as dichorionic-diamniotic, Sarah was confident that she wanted to have mostly midwifery-led care again but she would come into hospital this time for the births. However, in planning this approach Sarah came to realize that many midwives had not met with this request before, so she decided to move her care to another unit that had a neighbouring facility where she felt supported.

Progress throughout the pregnancy was normal and apart from increasing backache, Sarah approached her 37th week. A routine discussion was conducted in the clinic regarding the induction of labour for twin pregnancy, which normally is offered at 38 weeks gestation. Sarah of course had not experienced this intervention before and had always gone into spontaneous labour at around 40+12 days. She was keen to follow this route, as she felt this was better for herself and her unborn twins. Fetal growth was consistent, movements were normal and there was no sign of maternal disease at this point. Sarah agreed to come for weekly appointments until 41 weeks to ensure that these positive pregnancy markers continued.

At 41 weeks, Sarah had some signs of early labour with patterns of moderate painful but irregular contractions. A membrane sweep and induction of labour were discussed but once again Sarah was positive she would labour within 48 hours. As predicted by Sarah, she went into labour in the early evening and her first baby was born after a short labour in the cephalic position. The second twin converted from a cephalic position, which was maintained throughout pregnancy into a breech presentation. Wisely, the midwife waited and prepared for what she now knew was a breech presentation and after 35 minutes the breech presented and slowly birthed. The baby quickly cried, and was given skin-to-skin alongside his brother. The third stage was physiologically managed and the placentae were given to Sarah who planned their encapsulation.

Sarah had a short stay of 4 hours before going home to her waiting children to sleep in her own bed, with her mother and husband providing support until the community midwife visited the following morning.

Conclusion

What these two case studies demonstrate is that multiple pregnancy is a complex journey, although more often than not birth can be managed with some degree of maternal control. While families may be shocked upon confirmation of a multiple pregnancy, with midwifery support and input, it is possible to gain control and achieve birth events that provide both emotional and physical fulfilment.

Although the role of the midwife may not be as instrumental as with a routine low-risk woman, the emotional support that a midwife can provide is vitally important. Where women have difficult decisions to make, experience threats to the viability of their pregnancy and/or experience the death of one of the unborn babies, the midwife can be there to offer support over and beyond that normally given. It is those small gestures of kindness such as a phone call after a difficult appointment that make the difference. It is evident that support, kindness and compassion are key to midwifery care and especially where there are complex factors to pregnancies.

Useful websites

Multiple Births Foundation – an independent charity for families and professionals caring for multiple birth families; provides education, books, leaflets and other information [http://www.multiplebirths.org.uk/].

NHS Choices [www.nhs.uk/livewell/twins-and-multiples/pages/twins-and-multiples; www.nhs.uk/livewell/twins-and-multiples/pages/twins-facts; www.nhs.uk/Carersdirect].

Tamba – the Twins and Multiple Births Association (Tamba) is a registered charity set up by parents of twins, triplets and higher multiples and interested professionals [https://www.tamba.org.uk/].

Tamba's Bereavement Support Group [www.tamba-bsg.org.uk].

Twins Club – a website for parenting twins; find local twins club, chat with others, buy and sell equiptment [www.twinsclub.co.uk].

Twinsonline – for parents of twins and twins themselves from pregnancy to school age and beyond [www.twinsonline.org.uk].

Twin-to-Twin Transfusion Syndrome Association [www.twin2twin.org].

Twins UK – dedicated to families with twins, triplets and quads. Specialist products and information help make life with multiples easier and more enjoyable [www.twinsuk.co.uk].

References

Ballard, C.K., Bricker, L., Reed, K., Wood, L. and Neilson, J.P. (2011) Nutritional advice for improving outcomes in multiple pregnancies, *Cochrane Database of Systematic Reviews*, 6: CD008867.
Beemsterboer, S.N., Homburg, R., Gorter, N.A., Schats, R., Hompes, P.G. and Lambalk, C.B. (2006) The paradox of declining fertility but increasing twinning rates with advancing maternal age, *Human Reproduction*, 21 (6): 1531–2.
Bortolus, R., Fabio, P., Chatenoud, L., Benzi, G., Bianchi, M.M. and Marini, A. (1999) The epidemiology of multiple births, *Human Reproduction Update*, 5 (2): 179–87.
Bowlby, J. (1988) Attachment, communication, and the therapeutic process, in *A Secure Base: Parent child attachment and healthy human development*. London: Routledge.
Breathnach, F.M., McAuliffe, F.M., Geary, M., Daly, S., Higgins, J.R., Dornan, J. et al. (2011) Prediction of safe and successful vaginal twin birth, *American Journal of Obstetrics and Gynecology*, 205: 237.e1–7.
Caillagh, C. (2014) Coming to twins, *Midwifery Today*, 110 (Summer): 9–15.
Carrick-Sen, D.M., Steen, N. and Robson, S.C. (2014) Twin parenthood: the midwife's role – a randomised controlled trial, *BJOG: An International Journal of Obstetrics and Gynaecology*, 121 (10): 1302–10.
Chitayat, D. and Hall, J.G. (2006) Genetic aspects of twinning, in M. Kilby, P. Baker, H. Critchley and D. Field (eds) *Multiple Pregnancy*. London: RCOG Press.
Chung, K., Sammel, M.D., Coutifaris, C., Chalian, R., Lin, K., Castelbaum, A.J. et al. (2006) Defining the rise of serum HCG in viable pregnancies achieved through use of IVF, *Human Reproduction*, 21 (3): 823–8.
Dagustu, J. (2012) Beware the dead baby card, *AIMS Journal*, 24 (3).
Devaseelan, P. and Ong, S. (2010) Twin pregnancy: controversies in management, *The Obstetrician and Gynaecologist*, 12: 179–85.
Dodd, J.M., Crowther, C.A., Haslam, R.R. and Robinson, J.S. (2010) Timing of birth for women with a twin pregnancy at term: a randomised controlled trial, *BMC Pregnancy Childbirth*, 10: 68.
East, C.E., Dolan, W.J. and Forster, D.A. (2014) Antenatal breast milk expression by women with diabetes for improving infant outcomes, *Cochrane Database of Systematic Reviews*, 7: CD010408.

Eganhouse, D.J. and Petersen, L.A. (1998) Fetal surveillance in multifetal pregnancy, *Journal of Obstetric, Gynecologic, and Neonatal Nursing*, 27: 312–21.

Ekström, A., Thorstensson, S., Nilsson, M., Olsson, L. and Wahn, E.H. (2015) Women's experiences of midwifery support during pregnancy: a step in the validation of the scale: 'The Mother Perceived Support from Professionals', *Journal of Nursing and Care*, 4: 241.

Elbourne, D., Oakley, A. and Chalmers, I. (1989) Social and psychological support during pregnancy, in I. Chalmers, M.W. Enkin and M.J.N.C. Keirse (eds) *Effective Care in Pregnancy and Childbirth*. Oxford: Oxford University Press.

Fauser, B.C., Devroey, P. and Macklon, N.S. (2005) Multiple birth resulting from ovarian stimulation for subfertility treatment, *Lancet*, 365: 1807–16.

Fellman, J. and Eriksson, A.W. (2009) Statistical analyses of Hellin's law, *Twin Research and Human Genetics*, 12 (2): 191–200.

Fisk, N.M. (1995) The scientific basis of feto-fetal transfusion syndrome and its treatment, in H. Ward and M. Whittle (eds) *Proceedings of the RCOG Study Group on Multiple Pregnancy*. London: RCOG Press.

Gourheux, N., Deruelle, P., Houfflin-Debarge, V., Dubos, J.P. and Subtil, D. (2007) Intervalle de naissance entre les jumeaux: une limite de temps est-elle justifiée? [Twin-to-twin delivery interval: is a time limit justified?], *Gynécologie, Obstétrique et Fertilité*, 35: 982–9.

Gutteridge, K. (2013) MIDIRS Focus: Assessing progress through labour using midwifery wisdom, *Essentially MIDIRS*, 3 (3): 17–22.

Harper, L.M., Roehl, K., Odibo, A.O. and Cahill, A.G. (2013) First-trimester growth discordance and adverse pregnancy outcome in dichorionic twins, *Ultrasound in Obstetrics and Gynecology*, 41: 627–31.

Kitzinger, S. (2000) *Rediscovering Birth*. New York: Pocket Books.

Klaus, M., Kennell, J. and Klaus, P. (1995) *Bonding: Building the foundation of a secure attachment and independence*. Reading, MA: Addison-Wesley.

Lemay, G. (2002) Interventions, *Midwifery Today*, 63 (Autumn): 9.

Mitchell, L.M. (2004) Women's experiences of unexpected ultrasound findings, *Journal of Midwifery and Women's Health*, 49 (3): 228–34.

National Institute for Clinical Excellence (NICE) (2011) *Multiple Pregnancy: Antenatal care for twin and triplet pregnancies*, Clinical Guideline CG129. London: NICE [https://www.nice.org.uk/guidance/cg129].

National Institute for Clinical Excellence (NICE) (2013) *Multiple Pregnancy: Twin and triplet pregnancies*, Quality Standard QS46. London: NICE [https://www.nice.org.uk/guidance/qs46].

National Institute for Clinical Excellence (NICE) (2014) *Antenatal Care for Uncomplicated Pregnancies (2008): Review decision 2014*, Clinical Guideline CG62. London: NICE [https://www.nice.org.uk/guidance/cg62].

Newton, N. (1955) *Maternal Emotions*. New York: Paul Hober.

Newton, N., Foshee, D. and Newton, M. (1966) Parturient mice: effect of environment on labor, *Science*, 151 (3717): 1560–1.

Office for National Statistics (ONS) (2013) *Births in England and Wales by Characteristics of Birth 2: 2013*. London: ONS [http://www.ons.gov.uk/peoplepopulationand community/birthsdeathsandmarriages/livebirths/bulletins/characteristicsof birth2/2014-11-17].

Oleszczuk, J.J., Keith, D.M., Keith, L.G. and Rayburn, W.F. (1999) Projections of population-based twinning rates through the year 2100, *Journal of Reproductive Medicine*, 44 (11): 913–21.

Ozturk, O. and Templeton, A. (2002) *In-vitro* fertilisation and risk of multiple pregnancy, *Lancet,* 359 (9302): 232.

Parratt, J. and Fahy, K. (2011) A feminist critique of foundational nursing research and theory on transition to motherhood, *Midwifery,* 27 (4): 445–51.

Raphael-Leff, J. (2005) *Psychological Processes of Childbearing* (4th edn). London: Anna Freud Centre.

Rubin, R. (1975) Maternal tasks in pregnancy, *Maternal and Child Nursing Journal,* 4 (3): 143–53.

Schneuber, S., Magnet, E., Haas, J., Giuliani, A., Freidl, T., Lang, U. et al. (2011) Twin-to-twin delivery time: neonatal outcome of the second twin, *Twin Research and Human Genetics,* 14 (6): 573–9.

Skeie, A., Fröen, J.F., Vege, A. and Stray-Pedersen, B. (2003) Cause and risk of stillbirth in twin pregnancies: a retrospective audit, *Acta Obstetricia et Gynecologica Scandinavica,* 82 (11): 1010–16.

Smits, J. and Monden, C. (2011) Twinning across the developing world, *PLoS One,* 6 (9): e25239.

Thorpe, K., Golding, J., MacGivillivray, I. and Greenwood, R. (1991) Comparison of prevalence of depression in mothers of twins and mothers of singletons, *British Medical Journal,* 302: 875–8.

Utting, D. and Bewley, S. (2011) Family planning and age-related reproductive risk, *The Obstetrician and Gynaecologist,* 13: 25–41.

Walsh, D. and Gutteridge, K. (2011) Using the birth environment to increase women's potential in labour, *MIDIRS Midwifery Digest,* 21 (2): 143–7.

Ward Platt, M.P., Glinianaia, S.V., Rankin, J., Wright, C. and Renwick, M. (2006) The North of England Multiple Pregnancy Register: five-year results of data collection, *Twin Research and Human Genetics,* 9 (6): 913–18.

Williams, V. (2011) Is the 'high risk' label helpful?, *AIMS Journal,* 23 (4).

10

Vaginal birth after caesarean section
Helen Wightman

Introduction

In 1985, the World Health Organization (WHO) stated that rates of caesarean section above 10–15% conferred no reduction in maternal or neonatal morbidity or mortality, yet since this time there has been a steady rise in the rate of caesarean sections worldwide (Fioretti et al., 2014). Alongside this rise in the primary caesarean section rate, the incidence of vaginal birth after caesarean (VBAC) has declined in many countries recently (Bhide et al., 2013), contributing to the rising caesarean section rate. Reasons for these changes in primary mode of birth and the subsequent VBAC rate are multifactorial, complex and involve medical, human and social factors. In this chapter, I discuss some aspects of these factors and suggest a model of care to promote the provision of a VBAC service for women for whom there is no medical reason precluding a vaginal birth.

Background

In the United Kingdom, the caesarean section rate doubled between 1990 and 2008, with the rate being 26.2% in 2013. In 2010, the lowest European caesarean section rate was 14.8% in Iceland, with other countries including the Netherlands, Norway and Finland also achieving low rates (all under 20%) for both primary and repeat caesarean section. Cyprus had the highest rate at 52.2%, with several countries over 30%, including Germany, Italy and Portugal (Macfarlane et al., 2015).

Caesarean section rates worldwide have seen a similar upward trend, with figures reported to be over 50% in Brazil in 2010 (Guise et al., 2010) and 32.2% in the USA in 2014 (Childbirth Connection, 2015).

Impact of a caesarean birth

Although caesarean birth can be a life-saving event, it has the potential for adverse effects on both mother and baby. Compared with a vaginal birth, caesarean section has been estimated to more than double maternal mortality

(Landon et al., 2004). Early maternal morbidity complications such as haemorrhage, infection and the potential for hysterectomy, all require extended hospitalization and treatment (Chen and Hancock, 2012). Women also report significantly higher incidences of persistent pain following a caesarean birth (Kainu et al., 2010), with potential bladder and bowel injuries adding to the more long-term complications (Landon et al., 2004).

Neonatal complications include a higher risk of neonatal death, breathing problems due to transient tachypnoea, surgical injury and difficulties with breastfeeding (Villar et al., 2007; MacDorman et al., 2008; Zanardo et al., 2010). It is known that babies born vaginally are exposed to a wide variety of microbes, and differences in delivery mode have been linked to differences in the intestinal microbiota of babies. The relationship between the microbes is thought to benefit the maturation of the immune and intestinal system (Dominguez-Bello et al., 2010). The lack of fetal exposure to vaginal microbes during a caesarean birth is thought to make the baby more susceptible to certain pathogens. Dominguez-Bello et al. (2010) cite evidence that 64–82% of reported cases of babies with methicillin-resistant *Staphylococcus aureus* (MRSA) were born by caesarean section. Recent evidence has linked childhood obesity to maternal caesarean section, although some believe that this may be due to causal factors or reflect confounding influences (such as maternal obesity and reduced breastfeeding among mothers having a caesarean section) (Darmasseelane et al., 2014). Dominguez-Bello et al. (2010) also cite evidence that suggests babies born by caesarean are more prone to develop allergies and asthma. It is also acknowledged that little is known about the effects of caesarean birth on the long-term health of the child. Blustein and Liu (2015) have called for policy planning to include information regarding chronic illnesses in the child, as this may affect decision-making.

The impact on subsequent pregnancies includes a higher risk of stillbirth in the next pregnancy and an increased risk of postpartum haemorrhage (Kok et al., 2014). Other risks such as bladder, bowel and ureter injury, pelvic adhesions, the need for significant blood transfusion and an extended hospital stay are also significantly increased (Landon et al., 2004).

One of the most serious risks is placenta praevia and placenta accreta in subsequent pregnancies; its incidence has increased alongside the increase in the caesarean section rate, and is associated with significant maternal morbidity including peripartum hysterectomy (Paré et al., 2005). The continued rise in the primary caesarean section rate in parallel with falling VBAC rates will inevitably impact on these morbidities, with Paré et al. (2005) predicting that cases of placenta praevia and placenta accreta and associated morbidities will continue to rise.

Little is known about the long-term outcomes of a caesarean birth on both obstetric and gynaecological health and it is recognized that further research is needed in this area (Bhide et al., 2013).

Vaginal birth after caesarean section

Success rates for VBAC have been shown to be variable, ranging from 49 to 87% (Guise et al., 2010), with a decline reported in several countries; the success rate in the USA, for example, declined from 24% in 1996 to just 8% in 2010 (Knight et al., 2013). Knight et al. (2013) found that a little over 52% of UK women attempted a VBAC between 2004 and 2011, with approximately two-thirds of them achieving a successful vaginal birth. Variations between attempted and successful VBAC rates were also shown to exist between NHS trusts in the UK, suggesting that location impacts on choice and subsequent health outcomes.

The latest guideline of the Royal College of Obstetricians and Gynaecologists, 'Birth after Previous Caesarean Section' (RCOG, 2015), identifies a VBAC success rate of between 72 and 75%. Comparing this to Knight's data, it can reasonably be assumed that there exists a significant number of women who could achieve but do not attempt a VBAC. The original RCOG guidance for VBAC was published in 2007, with a similar predicted success rate for VBAC of 72–76%. Compared with Knight's data of an uptake of 52%, this brings into question the effectiveness of the national guidance in the years since 2007. One could argue that it is only guidance and not mandatory to follow, however, national guidance is based on current best available evidence and the rationale for not following best evidence should be made clear in the decision-making process.

Knight et al. (2013) acknowledge that little is known about rates of attempted VBAC in the UK, and that more detailed information regarding attempted and achieved VBAC, particularly in relation to geographical location and type of maternity unit, would provide women with more information to enhance their birth choices.

Impact on attitudes towards caesarean section

With the rise in the number of caesarean births, the perception of this method of birth has altered, and for many it is seen as 'normal' or a usual outcome of pregnancy. Traditionally, women have gained information about birth from experiential birth stories from other women (either positive or negative); Munro et al. (2009) found that narratives from women who had already undergone a caesarean birth served as encouragement to women when deciding whether to have the procedure themselves. Munro suggests that this will lead to a diminished knowledge of physiological birth resulting in a decrease in vaginal births.

Some women perceive a caesarean birth to be safer than a vaginal birth, despite the evidence clearly demonstrating that this is not the case (McCourt et al., 2007). Weaver (2000) found that women saw vaginal birth as risky and unpredictable, and considered caesarean birth a safe and routine alternative. With this familiarity comes the perception of safety, that the risks, although explained, have no bearing on the individual outcome due to the high incidence of the procedure. This leads one to question factors that impact and influence women; specifically, the quality, amount and methods of delivery of information to women, the perception of safety and the understanding and ability to apply risk during pregnancy.

Risk and how women interpret and balance risks and benefits will be discussed later in the chapter.

The benefits and risks of VBAC

It is important to note that the perinatal risks of a VBAC should be compared with those of a nulliparous women undergoing a first labour and should not be compared with those of an elective caesarean section, particularly when discussing the benefits and risks with women (Rozen et al., 2011; RCOG, 2015). Although there is thought to be little risk of a uterine rupture with an elective caesarean section, this is just one of the risks involved. Table 10.1 provides evidence of the benefits and risks of VBAC.

Factors affecting the success of an attempted VBAC

Table 10.2 provides details on relevant factors that might influence the decision to opt for a VBAC. The reported 40% success rate in Table 10.2 may influence women and they may prefer to undergo an elective caesarean rather than attempt a VBAC and then need an emergency caesarean. However, Kok et al. (2014) reported that the risk of stillbirth and postpartum haemorrhage was higher in the second birth following a primary elective than an emergency caesarean section, thus demonstrating that attempting a VBAC could be seen as a worthwhile undertaking, even if the chances of success are reduced.

   If a VBAC is unsuccessful, it is associated with lower maternal satisfaction and morbidities, including hysterectomy and operative complications (McMahon et al., 1996). These results were obtained when comparing VBAC criteria against a failed VBAC resulting in an emergency caesarean section; this highlights the importance of the RCOG (2015) recommendation that the risks of a VBAC be compared to that of a primigravida undergoing a first labour.

   No random controlled trials have been conducted comparing VBAC and repeat caesarean section, so decision-making can be a complex and difficult process. However, Brill and Windrim (2003) concluded that there are few absolute contraindications to attempt a VBAC, which brings into question the recent trend for an elective caesarean birth, with Kamal et al. (2005) describing the process as a 'social practice' with protocols having limited value.

Decision-making

The decision to choose an elective caesarean section or a VBAC is complex; perception of risk and maternal and neonatal safety, psychological, social and cultural factors have all been suggested to influence women's preferences (McCourt et al., 2007). The assessment, communication and management of risk have been described as one of the most challenging tasks in medicine, often leading to detrimental care that is not women-centred or evidence-based (Lyerly et al., 2007). Lyerly also highlighted the ethical complexities of decision-making for repeat caesarean section or VBAC, acknowledging that safety and women's autonomy against the backdrop of the increasing caesarean birth rate contributes to the decision.

Table 10.1 The risks and benefits of VBAC.

Benefits	Risks
• VBAC results in a quicker postpartum recovery, leading to reduced hospital stays, which reduces costs (Schoorel et al., 2013). • Physical complications associated with a caesarean birth detailed previously will be avoided. • Women who have achieved a VBAC report high levels of satisfaction (Dunn and O'Herlihy, 2005). • Early contact with the newborn, specifically within the context of the relationship between bonding and successful breastfeeding (Meddings et al., 2007). • Women achieving a vaginal birth hold their baby for longer, are more likely to successfully initiate breastfeeding and are more likely to breastfeed upon discharge. These aspects have been shown to influence women's decision-making when considering caesarean section or VBAC (Meddings et al., 2007; Regan et al., 2013; Redshaw et al., 2014). • Women who have experienced both caesarean section and a vaginal birth favour vaginal birth in subsequent pregnancies. This may be because women perceive a vaginal birth to be associated with a quicker recovery in the postpartum period (Eden et al., 2005). • Women who strongly favour a VBAC see it as the best start in life for their baby and a significant life event for themselves (Phillips et al., 2009). • A VBAC is more cost-effective than a caesarean section, with estimates that a caesarean section is approximately 44% more expensive than a vaginal birth. These costs associated with a caesarean section become cumulative, due to the number of repeat caesarean births (Allen et al., 2006; Fawsitt et al., 2013; Petrou and Khan, 2013).	• Uterine rupture can potentially lead to a neonatal death and the associated maternal mortality or morbidity. The specific risk of uterine rupture has been estimated as 0.5%, or 1 per 200 births, although rates have been shown to vary depending on onset of labour (RCOG, 2015). • Postpartum haemorrhage and hysterectomy (RCOG, 2015).

Table 10.2 Factors affecting an attempted VBAC.

Factors known to improve the likelihood of achieving a VBAC	Factors known to reduce the likelihood of a successful VBAC
Previous vaginal birth; if this has been achieved, then the success rate for a VBAC is estimated at 85–90%.	No previous vaginal birth.
Body mass index below 30.	Body mass index greater than 30.
A spontaneous labour will increase the potential for a VBAC, with the incidence of uterine rupture decreased if a previous VBAC has been achieved.	Induced labour, no previous vaginal birth, BMI greater than 30 and previous caesarean for labour dystocia, together reduce the likelihood of a successful VBAC to 40%.
White ethnicity.	Non-white ethnicity.
Maternal age below 40 years.	Advanced maternal age.
Infant birth weight below 4 kg.	Infant birth weight above 4 kg.
Pregnancy before 41 weeks gestation.	Pregnancy after 41 weeks gestation.
Vertex presentation, fetal head engagement and a higher admission Bishop score.	Cervical dilatation less than 4 cm on hospital admission in labour.
More likely in women who had previous caesarean for fetal malposition than either cervical dystocia or fetal distress. Of those with cervical dystocia, more likely if cervical dilatation reaches 8 cm.	Previous preterm caesarean birth.
Previous caesarean for failed forceps birth.	Previous failed induction of labour.

Source: RCOG (2015).

Consideration and perception of risk

Decision-making is often made alongside a consideration of risk. Women can be fearful and anxious when faced with the decision regarding mode of birth and some women describe a sense of relief if the decision is made for them, as it prevents feelings of guilt regarding the decision (Shorten et al., 2014). However, being involved in decision-making can also contribute to a feeling of control, an important factor for some women (Lundgren et al., 2012), as well as increased trust in those involved in their care (Meddings et al., 2007). Some women, however, do not like being involved in the decision (Gamble and Creedy, 2001) or may question their decision after the birth (Emmett et al., 2006). Women sometimes do not want to risk another emergency caesarean birth, preferring the certainty of an elective caesarean, often with family commitments in mind (Meddings et al., 2007). This may be the case even if they are strong candidates for VBAC, with some women thought to be displaying altruism, engaging in the risks of a caesarean section for the sake of the baby so that they are not seen to be selfish. Previous childbirth experiences can have a powerful effect on the decision, with safety of the baby often paramount (Eden et al., 2004; Shorten et al., 2014). Choice and decision-making by women can also lead to uncertainty, resulting in a change of place of birth or lead clinician (Lundgren et al., 2012).

Many biases exist in the way risk is conceptualized and interpreted, with many people having difficulty interpreting numerical information that could lead to overreliance on 'inviduating information', for example, anecdotal information (Kaimal and Kuppermann, 2010). Also, the risk dialogue in pregnancy regarding probabilities is often undertaken without any consideration of women's values or prioritizing the reduction of risk to the fetus (Lyerly et al., 2007), although Eden et al. (2005) found that women prioritized the safety of their baby four times more than their own safety. However, women are not always fully aware of the benefits and risks of VBAC (Chen and Hancock, 2012), which in itself could be seen to be restricting their choices.

The perceived severity of a condition affects decision-making. Women who are strongly in favour of a VBAC have been found to display a higher internal locus of control than those choosing another caesarean; these women may also be influenced more by online sources than healthcare professionals (Konheim-Kalkstein et al., 2014). Increased knowledge about the risks and benefits of both repeat caesarean section and VBAC has been shown to increase the number of women opting for a VBAC (Scaffadi et al., 2014).

Women's perception of difficulties might prevent a successful VBAC. McGrath et al. (2010, cited in Lundgren et al., 2012) found that some women perceived that they did not have a real choice of giving birth vaginally based on the risk of uterine rupture.

Dahlen and Homer (2013) investigated women's perception of risk on inter-net blog sites and discovered they often discussed whether or not they were under- or overestimating the risk involved. The authors also noted that when approaching decision-making regarding mode of birth, women either put the baby first (so-called 'childbirth') or took the view that birthing naturally resulted in a happier mother, and thus a happier child (so-called 'motherbirth'). Women clearly have different perspectives to clinicians on factors that are important to their decision-making, demonstrating that no 'one size fits all'.

Although some women are influenced more by online information (Konheim-Kalkstein et al., 2014), evidence suggests that this information may not be complete. Many popular websites favour repeat caesarean section, do not provide the best available evidence or are aimed at an academic audience, thus making the information presented there difficult to understand (Fioretti et al., 2014; Whitelaw et al., 2014; Bantan and Abenheim, 2015). Chen and Hancock (2012) discovered that most women are aware that a caesarean section is considered major surgery but a significant proportion are unaware of potential complications for the baby or themselves.

Moffat et al. (2006) found that women's feelings about the quality and amount of information they received regarding mode of birth varied a great deal; standard information regarding benefits and risks was not always helpful, with many women wanting the information to be tailored to their individual circumstances.

It is recommended that discussion of the risks, benefits and implications of birth by caesarean section or VBAC leads to a shared decision between the woman and the healthcare provider (RCOG, 2015). To aid this process, prediction models have been developed to provide further information to women regarding their individual risks and the potential for success (Schoorel et al., 2013).

Maternal satisfaction surrounding decision-making has been linked to the amount of information received (Renner et al., 2007). The recognition of the different approaches to decision-making has led to the creation of a range of decision-making aids for women (Shorten et al., 2005; Emmett et al., 2006; Montgomery et al., 2007; Schoorel et al., 2013). These aim to provide information and tailor individual risk factors in an attempt to provide clear and comprehensive information in an unbiased way.

Some of these aids, however, focus on the clinical facts surrounding caesarean birth and VBAC and do not take into consideration health beliefs, women's expectation of childbirth or their individual family circumstances. Farnworth et al. (2008) recognize that there are often complex emotional and social factors that impact on the decision to be taken. Family obligations towards other siblings related to postpartum recovery have been cited to be important for women when considering VBAC (Meddings et al., 2007). Cultural beliefs about the birthing process have also been found to affect women's perceptions of a caesarean birth (Hsu et al., 2008), and have an impact on the rates of caesarean section as discussed earlier in the chapter.

Schoorel et al. (2013) believe tailored, structured individual information to be the best aid for women in their decision-making, and recognize that the aids might bring about clinician consensus regarding medical facts. However, it could be seen that providing 'tailored and structured' information to women might not fulfil the need for clinicians to provide full and unbiased information to facilitate informed choice.

Montgomery et al. (2007) found that using a decision aid could add to the uncertainty of decision-making, and Lyerly et al. (2007) describe how the non-directive choices designed to promote autonomy sometimes leave women feeling abandoned and less informed. However, some women use the information gained through the decision-making aid as a starting point to look for more information (Frost et al., 2009).

Shorten et al. (2005) found that a decision aid tool increased women's level of knowledge and decreased decisional conflict, but concluded that there was little evidence that this led to informed choice. This suggests that providing effective informed choice in conjunction with shared decision-making, although often cited as best practice, does not necessarily occur. In line with Horey et al. (2013), Nilsson et al. (2015) concluded that although decision aids do not affect the VBAC rate, they provide information regarding mode of birth and overall reduce decisional conflict.

The concept of risk is discussed in detail in Chapter 3.

Health professionals

The concept of choice has been a focus in healthcare and specifically childbirth since the early 1990s, and facilitating informed choice is an important part of the role of the healthcare professional (Department of Health, 1993; NICE, 2011; RCOG, 2015).

The views of the clinician can exert a strong influence on the decision taken by women, and the women are not always given all the information regarding elective caesarean and VBAC. The mode of delivery suggested is sometimes aligned more with the workings of the specific institution than the women's preferences (Shorten et al., 2005; Bernstein et al., 2012). This is particularly apparent in countries with higher rates of private healthcare; for example, Guise et al. (2010) found that choices regarding mode of birth following a previous caesarean sometimes result from non-medical factors such as clinician preference, concerns about medical liability or hospital policy.

Health professionals are sometimes seen as helping unravel conflicting or contradictory information (Lundgren et al., 2012); however there is substantial evidence of inconsistency of clinician opinions, women often see different doctors during pregnancy thereby potentially adding to their confusion.

Health professionals will be guided by national guidelines, although Foureur et al. (2010) have questioned their value. In considering the evidence used in six sets of national guidelines published between 2004 and 2007, Foureur and colleagues found significant differences between them, including reported success rates, risks of uterine rupture, the use of continuous electronic fetal monitoring and induction of labour. With such diversity of guidelines between western countries, it is evident that providing robust guidance for women and healthcare professionals is a problem, especially when local policy is determined by this guidance.

Many women have already formed an opinion regarding mode of birth before they attend for antenatal care (Dodd et al., 2013). Providing women with information leaflets is recommended by RCOG (2015), although these often provide clinical information only – it is thus important that women's values and feelings are included in all discussions with clinicians. This therefore relies on the clinician respecting and following guidance on shared decision-making and strengthens the need to observe national strategies for schedules of antenatal care to promote safe and appropriate VBAC (RCOG, 2015).

This leads to conjecture around the amount and quality of information that women receive from health professionals, as women need to be given information not only regarding the risks but also the benefits of VBAC, and in the context of their individual circumstances. Scioscia et al. (2008) make a valuable point that with so many factors involved in decision-making, a simple policy is unlikely to be effective; instead, any policy needs to encompass the opinions of women and not just be a declaration of intent of shared decision-making. Monari et al. (2008) investigated midwives' and obstetricians' personal attitudes towards caesarean section, and found that midwives were more concerned with the risks of that procedure and more likely to support women requesting a VBAC. Information-sharing and counselling of women by all healthcare professionals need to be unbiased, thorough and have relevance to women's personal values and situations.

Recently, educational intervention projects with healthcare professionals have been introduced in both Canada and Spain with the aim of improving quality and safety by decreasing unnecessary repeat caesarean sections (Bermúdez-Tamayo et al., 2014). Research from Portugal (Ayres-de-Campos et al., 2015) describes a recent reduction in the national caesarean section rate and an improvement in the VBAC rate after the government introduced a policy aimed at reducing caesarean sections. This comprised education of healthcare profession-als and changes in hospital funding. Alongside the reduced caesarean section rate and increased VBAC rate, perinatal mortality rate was also decreased. The evi-dence from Portugal demonstrates that it is possible to halt and then reverse the trend for caesarean section, although it remains to be seen whether this trend continues and other countries adopt such a positive attitude as Portugal.

Finally, an effective shared decision-making model with women at its centre would ensure that decision-making is based on informed consent. Healthcare pro-fessionals need to set aside personal feelings and bias and understand and com-municate the evidence regarding VBAC in a supportive and non-judgemental way. Robust methods of audit are needed to record the attempted and actual VBAC rates, which in turn will add to women's choices and provide institutions with data to subsequently inform and improve evidence-based care.

Moving forward

Nilsson et al. (2015) identified an urgent need to develop woman-centred interven-tions to help improve VBAC rates. Changes in the organization and 'hierarchical structures' within maternity services to embed midwifery-led models of care may help reduce caesarean section rates and improve the uptake of VBAC (Gamble et al., 2007). Lundgren et al. (2015) evaluated clinician-centred interventions aimed at increasing the uptake of VBAC and found limited research in this area. However, they did identify that clinician-centred interventions needed to relate to a coun-try's culture and maternity care settings. Midwifery-led models of care are asso-ciated with improved outcomes for women (Hatem et al., 2008), and dedicated clinics specifically for women who have had a previous caesarean section have been positively evaluated for their impact on VBAC rates (Gardner et al., 2014). Knowledge and appreciation of the many dimensions that inform women's decision-making have been found to be important when considering VBAC services (Fenwick et al., 2007). A project to improve the organization of maternal health service delivery by increasing VBAC through enhancing women-centred care is currently being conducted, with completion expected in 2016 (Begley, 2013).

A midwife-led VBAC service

Within a climate of increasing high-risk pregnancies, it could be argued that one previous caesarean section with no other risk factors no longer considers a second pregnancy to be high risk. As midwives have been found to be more likely to sup-port a VBAC, it seems natural to provide a midwife-led service for women who have had one previous caesarean section with no other risk factors.

There are several UK health services in which women who have had one cae-sarean section but who are otherwise low risk, follow an antenatal pathway led by midwives (Barnes, 2010). The women, who are identified at booking at approxi-mately 8–12 weeks gestation and are reviewed by one or two specialist midwives, are able to discuss their choices for mode of birth; this pathway promotes consistency of information, continuity of care and collaboration between professional groups as appropriate. A risk assessment at booking highlights any women that need obstetric referral. Next, the women are reviewed by an obstetrician at 12–14 weeks gestation, with a VBAC encouraged if there has been just one previous caesarean birth. An initial plan is documented by 20 weeks gestation and a final plan is made by 36 weeks gestation, with further obstetric review at 41 weeks gestation if labour has not occurred spontaneously. Women who choose an elective repeat caesarean section are accommodated appropriately.

The financial benefits associated with a reduced caesarean section rate and improved short- and long-term health benefits need to be collated through robust audit procedures. Regular multi-professional education and feedback can be used as an effective tool to promote a reduction in the caesarean section rate and improve VBAC uptake.

Case 10.1: Lisa

Lisa had her first baby by caesarean section for a breech presentation at 38 weeks gestation. Lisa did not want a repeat caesarean section for her second birth, as she had a toddler to care for. She did not want any antenatal parentcraft education, she was aware of the recommendation for continuous electronic fetal monitoring for her labour, and was aware of her options during labour – however, she was not aware of the option of water immersion for labour and the possibility of water birth.

Upon arrival at the hospital in the early hours of the morning, Lisa's cervix was found to be 5 cm dilated; she was coping well with the contractions. The senior labour suite midwife was known to be a strong supporter of optimizing normal birth, so the midwife caring for Lisa felt confident in autonomously offering Lisa the option of the pool for labour, in a pool room located on the 'consultant-led' side of the labour suite. Lisa readily accepted the pool option; indeed, the impression from the attending midwife was that Lisa viewed this as 'normal' care. The labour room was adapted to give it a more 'home-like' feel, with low lighting, music and a birthing mat, with one-to-one care given by the experienced midwife.

Lisa immediately relaxed when entering the pool, and had continuous fetal monitoring using a telemetry cardiotocograph. The midwife did not offer Lisa a venous cannula, as she judged that Lisa had peripheral veins that would be easy to cannulate in an emergency and Lisa was not anaemic. The midwife was aware that the risk of uterine rupture is comparable to that of a cord prolapse and that women are not routinely advised to have a venous cannula in labour 'just in case' the cord might prolapse; however, she also judged that Lisa was haemodynamically stable and did not show any signs of uterine rupture.

The second stage of labour commenced after Lisa had been in the pool for about 90 minutes. Baby Ben was born 30 minutes later. The placenta delivered physiologically (this was unplanned).

The midwife caring for Lisa was particularly proud of this moment in her career, as it was one of the first water VBACs to be carried out in the unit and she was able to facilitate a good birth experience for Lisa. The interprofessional trust between midwives and obstetricians enabled a rational clinical decision to be made regarding a cannula, and the environment of the labour room provided a relaxed atmosphere for Lisa.

On discussion with Lisa after the birth, it transpired that Lisa was unaware that she was considered high risk; she said that she had been told that she would be 'strapped to the bed' but she didn't really understand why she was considered high risk. She reported that when the midwife offered her the pool and she saw how the room was set up, she assumed that all VBAC women were offered the pool for labour or birth, that this was usual practice. She also commented positively on the midwive's attitude, that she didn't 'make a fuss' and she 'let her get on with it'.

Practice points

- How does your own high-risk labour suite area promote an environment that is conducive to privacy, relaxation and a positive birth experience? What simple and cost-effective improvements could be made to 'high-risk' areas that would promote the physiological labour process?
- How can midwives and obstetricians work together to promote the uptake of VBAC by women?
- Could a specific midwife-led model of antenatal care for women with no other obstetric risk factors be implemented for VBAC?
- Consider your own knowledge regarding VBAC. Do you feel sufficiently knowledgeable to converse with women, their families and inter-professionally to provide the facts that would support a true informed choice?

Case 10.2: Eleanor

Eleanor had a previous caesarean section for 'cervical dystocia' towards the end of the first stage of labour and was very keen to achieve a VBAC with her second birth. Staff worked with her and her husband to promote her choices in labour, and a high-risk labour room was adapted to appear more like a low-risk room. However, a telemetry cardiotocograph (CTG) was unavailable, so Eleanor's mobility in active labour was limited to the length of the wires on the so-called 'normal' CTG. This proved difficult due to loss of contact. Eleanor did not wish to have a fetal scalp electrode applied and eventually removed the CTG altogether, as she wished to remain mobile in labour. The midwife made clear to Eleanor the policy and advice regarding continuous fetal monitoring but Eleanor was adamant that she needed to remain mobile. Following this conversation, the midwife observed that Eleanor relaxed, became less communicative and labour advanced well. Later, after a change of shifts by the midwives, Eleanor did consent to electronic fetal monitoring and had a vacuum birth due to a pathological CTG.

The first midwife caring for Eleanor was able to discuss her labour with Eleanor the following day; Eleanor was exceptionally pleased that she had achieved a vaginal birth. Eleanor reported that she felt very strongly that she needed to remain mobile in labour; she felt that the reason she had 'failed' in her first labour was because she was strapped to the bed. She also felt extra pressure in the current pregnancy because she had been labelled 'high risk'.

Practice points

- Does your maternity unit offer telemetry CTG?
- How can midwives impact financial decision-making so that effective care can be maximized for high-risk labours to then provide cost efficiencies in the longer term?
- Does the attitude of the multi-professional team ensure that women are treated as individuals and autonomy is not only promoted but also respected? How can midwives safely support women's choices when faced with a situation like Eleanor's?
- Do women in your care receive sufficient information regarding options for VBAC and do professionals assume that this has been addressed thoroughly before the start of labour?

Further reading

McKenna, J.A. and Symon, A.G. (2013) Water VBAC: exploring a new frontier for women's autonomy, *Midwifery*, 30: e20–35. Provides a discussion of waterbirth VBAC within the context of choice and autonomy.

Vadeboncoeur, H. (2011) *Birthing Normally After a Caesarean or Two*. Chester-le-Street: Fresh Heart Publishing. Provides an in-depth discussion of VBAC and suggests practical help and support for both women and midwives.

Useful websites

AIMS – Association for Improvements in the Maternity Services [www.aims.org.uk].

ARM – Association of Radical Midwives [www.radmid.demon.co.uk].

NCT – National Childbirth Trust [www.nct.org.uk].

RCM – Royal College of Midwives [www.rcm.org.uk].

RCOG – Royal College of Obstetricians and Gynaecologists [www.rcog.org.uk].

References

Allen, V.M., O'Connell, C.M. and Baskett, T.F. (2006) Cumulative economic implications of initial method of delivery, *Obstetrics and Gynecology*, 108 (3 Pt. 1): 549–55.

Ayres-de-Campos, D., Cruz, J., Medeiros-Borges, C., Costa-Santos, C. and Vicente, L. (2015) Lowered national caesarean section rates after a concerted action, *Acta Obstetricia Gynecologica Scandinavica*, 94 (4): 391–8.

Bantan, N. and Abenheim, H.A. (2015) Vaginal births after caesarean: what does Google think about it?, *Women and Birth*, 28 (1): 21–4.

Barnes, H. (2010) Midwife-led antenatal care for women with a previous caesarean section, *MIDIRS Midwifery Digest*, 20 (1): 41–5.

Begley, C. (2013) *Improving the Organisation of Maternal Health Service Delivery, and Optimising Childbirth, by Increasing Vaginal Birth after Caesarean Section (VBAC) through Enhanced Women-centred Care* [http://www.isrctn.com/ISRCTN10612254; accessed 22 April 2015].

Bermúdez-Tamayo, C., Johri, M., Perez-Ramos, F.J., Maroto-Navarro, G., Cano-Aguilar, A., Garcia-Mochon, L. et al. (2014) Evaluation of quality improvement for cesarean section programmes through mixed methods, *Implementation Science*, 9: 182.

Bernstein, S.N., Matalon-Grazi, S. and Rosenn, B.M. (2012) Trial of labour versus repeat cesarean: are patients making an informed decision?, *American Journal of Obstetrics and Gynecology*, 207 (3): 204.e1–6.

Bhide, A., Jauniaux, E. and Silver, B. (2013) BJOG Editors' Choice, *BJOG: An International Journal of Obstetrics and Gynaecology*, 121 (2): i–ii.

Blustein, J. and Liu, J. (2015) Time to consider the risks of caesarean delivery for long term child health, *British Medical Journal*, 350: h2410.

Brill, Y. and Windrim, R. (2003) Vaginal birth after caesarean section: review of antenatal predictors of success, *Journal of Obstetrics and Gynaecology Canada*, 25 (4): 275–86.

Chen, M.M. and Hancock, H. (2012) Women's knowledge of options for birth after caesarean section, *Women and Birth*, 25 (3): e19–26.

Childbirth Connection (2015) *Cesarean Section*. Washington, DC: National Partnership for Women and Families [http://www.childbirthconnection.org/article.asp?ck=10554; accessed 22 April 2015].

Dahlen, H.G. and Homer, C.S.E. (2013) Motherbirth or childbirth? A prospective analysis of vaginal birth after caesarean blogs, *Midwifery*, 29 (2): 167–73.

Darmasseelane, K., Hyde, M.J., Santhakumaran, S., Gale, C. and Modi, N. (2014) Mode of delivery and offspring body mass index, overweight and obesity in adult life: a systematic review and meta-analysis, *PLoS One*, 9 (2): e87896.

Department of Health (1993) *Changing Childbirth: Report of the Expert Maternity Group*. London: HMSO.

Dodd, J.M., Crowther, C.A., Huertas, E., Guise, J.M. and Horey, D. (2013) Planned elective repeat caesarean versus planned vaginal birth for women with a previous caesarean birth (review), *Cochrane Database of Systematic Reviews*, 12: CD004224.

Dominguez-Bello, M.G., Costello, E.K., Contreras, M., Magris, M., Hidalgo, G., Fierer, N. et al. (2010) Delivery mode shapes the acquisition and structure of the initial microbiota across multiple body habitats in newborns, *Proceedings of the National Academy of Sciences USA*, 107 (26): 11971–5.

Dunn, E.A. and O'Herlihy, C. (2005) Comparison of maternal satisfaction following vaginal delivery after caesarean section and caesarean section after previous vaginal delivery, *European Journal of Obstetrics & Gynecology and Reproductive Biology*, 121 (21): 56–60.

Eden, K.B., Dolan, J.G., Perrin, N.A., Kocaoglu, D., Anderson, N., Case, J. et al. (2005) Patients were more consistent in randomized trial at prioritizing childbirth preferences using graphic-numeric than verbal formats, *Journal of Clinical Epidemiology*, 62 (4): 415–24.

Eden, K.B., Hashima, J.N., Osterweil, P., Nygren, P. and Guise, J.M. (2004) Childbirth preferences after cesarean birth: a review of the evidence, *Birth*, 31 (1): 49–60.

Emmett, C.L., Shaw, A.R.G., Montgomery, A.A., Murphy, D.J. and DiAMOND study group (2006) Women's experience of decision making about mode of delivery after a previous caesarean section: the role of health professionals and information about health risks, *BJOG: An International Journal of Obstetrics and Gynaecology*, 113 (12): 1438–45.

Farnworth, A., Robson, S.C., Thomson, R.G., Watson, D.B. and Murtagh, M.J. (2008) Decision support for women choosing mode of delivery after a previous caesarean section: a developmental study, *Patient Education and Counselling*, 71 (1): 116–24.

Fawsitt, C.G., Bourke, J., Greene, R.A., Everard, C.M., Murphy, A. and Lutomski, J.E. (2013) At what price? A cost-effectiveness analysis comparing trial of labour versus elective repeat caesarean delivery, *PLoS One*, 8 (3): e58577.

Fenwick, J., Gamble, J. and Hauck, Y. (2007) Believing in birth-choosing VBAC: the childbirth expectations of a self-selected cohort of Australian women, *Journal of Clinical Nursing*, 16 (8): 1561–70.

Fioretti, B.T.S., Reiter, M., Betrán, A.P. and Torloni, M.R. (2014) Googling caesarean section: a survey on the quality of the information available on the Internet, *BJOG: An International Journal of Obstetrics and Gynaecology*, 122 (5): 731–9.

Foureur, M., Ryan, C., Nicholl, M. and Homer, C. (2010) Inconsistent evidence: analysis of six national guidelines for vaginal birth after cesarean section, *Birth*, 37 (1): 3–10.

Frost, J., Shaw, A., Montgomery, A. and Murphy, D.J. (2009) Women's views on the use of decision aids for decision making about the method of delivery following a previous caesarean section: qualitative interview study, *BJOG: An International Journal of Obstetrics and Gynaecology*, 116 (7): 896–905.

Gamble, J.A. and Creedy, D.K. (2001) Women's preference for a caesarean section: incidence and associated factors, *Birth*, 28 (2): 101–10.

Gamble, J.A., Creedy, D.K., McCourt, C., Weaver, J. and Beake, S. (2007) A critique of the literature on women's request for caesarean section: incidence and associated factors, *Birth*, 34 (4): 331–40.

Gardner, K., Henry, A., Thou, S., Davis, G. and Miller, T. (2014) Improving VBAC rates: the combined impact of two management strategies, *Australian and New Zealand Journal of Obstetrics and Gynaecology*, 54 (4): 327–32.

Guise, J.M., Eden, K., Emeis, C., Denman, M.A., Marshall, N., Fu, R.R. et al. (2010) Vaginal birth after cesarean: new insights, *Evidence Report/Technology Assessment*, 191: 1–397.

Hatem, M., Sandall, J., Devane, D., Soltani, H. and Gates, G. (2008) Midwifery-led versus other models of care for childbearing women, *Cochrane Database of Systematic Reviews*, 4: CD004667.

Horey, D., Kealy, M., Davey, M.A., Small, R. and Crowther, C.A. (2013) Interventions for supporting women's decision-making about mode of birth after a caesarean, *Cochrane Database of Systematic Reviews*, 7: CD010041.

Hsu, K.H., Lioa, P.J. and Hwang, C.J. (2008) Factors affecting Taiwanese women's choice of caesarean section, *Social Science and Medicine*, 66 (1): 201–9.

Kaimal, A.J. and Kuppermann, M. (2010) Understanding risk, patient and provider preferences, and obstetrical decision making: approach to delivery after caesarean, *Seminars in Perinatology*, 34 (5): 331–6.

Kainu, J.P., Halmesmäki, E. and Korttila, K.T. (2010) Persistent pain after caesarean section and vaginal birth: a cohort study, *International Journal of Obstetric Anesthesia*, 19 (1): 4–9.

Kamal, P., Dixon-Woods, M., Kurinczuk, J., Oppenheimer, C., Squire, P. and Waugh, J. (2005) Factors influencing repeat caesarean section: qualitative exploratory study of obstetricians' and midwives' accounts, *BJOG: An International Journal of Obstetrics and Gynaecology*, 112 (8): 1054–60.

Knight, H.E., Gurol-Urganci, I., van der Meulen, J.H., Mahmood, T.A., Richmond, D.H., Dougall, A. et al. (2013) Vaginal birth after caesarean section: a cohort study investigating factors associated with its uptake and success, *BJOG: An International Journal of Obstetrics and Gynaecology*, 121 (2): 183–93.

Kok, N., Ruiter, L., Hof, M., Ravelli, A., Mol, B.W., Pajkrt, E. et al. (2014) Risk of maternal and neonatal complications in subsequent pregnancy after planned caesarean section in a first birth, compared with emergency caesarean section: a nationwide comparative cohort study, *BJOG: An International Journal of Obstetrics and Gynaecology*, 121 (2): 216–23.

Konheim-Kalkstein, Y.L., Barry, M.M. and Galotti, K. (2014) Examining influences on women's decision to try labour after previous caesarean section, *Journal of Reproductive and Infant Psychology*, 32 (2): 137–47.

Landon, M.B., Hauth, J.C., Leveno, K.J., Spong, C.Y., Leindecker, S., Varner, M.W. et al. (2004) Maternal and perinatal outcomes associated with a trial of labor after prior cesarean delivery, *New England Journal of Medicine*, 351 (25): 2581–9.

Lundgren, I., Begley, C., Gross, M.M. and Bondas, T. (2012) 'Groping through the fog': a metasynthesis of women's experiences on VBAC (vaginal birth after caesarean section), *BMC Pregnancy and Childbirth*, 12: 85.

Lundgren, I., Smith, V., Nilsson, C., Vehvilainen-Julkunen, K., Nicoletti, J., Devane, D. et al. (2015) Clinician-centred interventions to increase vaginal birth after caesarean section (VBAC): a systematic review, *BMC Pregnancy and Childbirth*, 15: 16.

Lyerly, A.D., Mitchell, L.M., Armstrong, E.M., Harris, L.H., Kukla, R., Kuppermann, M. et al. (2007) Risks, values and decision making surrounding pregnancy, *Obstetrics and Gynecology*, 109 (4): 979–84.

MacDorman, M.F., Declercq, E., Menacker, F. and Malloy, M.H. (2008) Neonatal mortality for primary cesarean and vaginal births to low-risk women: application of an 'intention-to-treat' model, *Birth*, 35 (1): 3–8.

Macfarlane, A.J., Blondel, B., Mohangoo, A.D., Cuttini, M., Nijhuis, J., Novak, Z. et al. (2015) Wide differences in mode of delivery within Europe: risk-stratified analyses of aggregated routine data from the Euro-Peristat study. *BJOG: An International Journal of Obstetrics and Gynaecology*, 123 (4): 559–68.

McCourt, C., Weaver, J., Statham, H., Beake, S., Gamble, J. and Creedy, D.K. (2007) Elective cesarean section and decision making: a critical review of the literature. *Birth*, 34 (1): 65–79.

McGrath, P., Philips, E. and Vaughan, G. (2010) Speaking out! Qualitative insights on the experiences of mothers who wanted a vaginal birth after birth by caesarean section, *Patient*, 3 (1): 25–32.

McMahon, M.J., Edwin, R., Luther, M.D., Watson, A., Bowes, M.D. and Olshan, A.F. (1996) Comparison of a trial of labor with an elective second cesarean section, *New England Journal of Medicine*, 335 (10): 689–95.

Meddings, F., MacVane Philips, F., Haith-Cooper, M. and Haigh, J. (2007) Vaginal birth after caesarean section (VBAC): exploring women's perceptions, *Journal of Clinical Nursing*, 16 (1): 160–7.

Moffat, M.A., Bell, J.S., Porter, M.A., Lawton, S., Hundley, V., Danielian, P. et al. (2006) Decision making about mode of delivery among pregnant women who have previously had a caesarean section: a qualitative study, *BJOG: An International Journal of Obstetrics and Gynaecology*, 114 (1): 86–93.

Monari, F., Di Mario, S., Facchinetti, F. and Basevi, V. (2008) Obstetricians' and midwives' attitudes toward caesarean section, *Birth*, 35 (2): 129–35.

Montgomery, A.A., Emmett, C.L., Fahey, T., Jones, C., Ricketts, I., Patel, R.R. et al. (2007) Two decision aids for mode of delivery among women with previous caesarean section: randomised controlled trial, *British Medical Journal*, 334 (7607): 1305.

Munro, S., Kornelsen, J. and Hutton, E. (2009) Decision making in patient-initiated elective cesarean delivery: the influence of birth stories, *Journal of Midwifery and Women's Health*, 54 (5): 373–9.

National Institute for Health and Clinical Excellence (NICE) (2011) *Caesarean Section*, Clinical Guideline CG132. London: NICE [https://www.nice.org.uk/guidance/cg132; accessed 22 April 2015].

Nilsson, C., Lundgren, I., Smith, V., Vehvilainen-Julkunen, K., Nicoletti, J., Devane, D. et al. (2015) Woman-centred interventions to increase vaginal birth after caesarean section (VBAC): a systematic review, *Midwifery*, 31 (7): 657–63.

Paré, E., Quinones, J.N. and Macones, G.A. (2005) Vaginal birth after caesarean versus elective repeat caesarean section: assessment of maternal downstream health outcomes, *BJOG: An International Journal of Obstetrics and Gynaecology*, 113 (1): 75–85.

Petrou, S. and Khan, K. (2013) An overview of the health economic implications of elective caesarean section, *Applied Health Economics and Health Policy*, 11 (6): 561–76.

Phillips, E., McGrath, P. and Vaughan, G. (2009) 'I wanted desperately to have a natural birth': mothers' insights on vaginal birth after caesarean (VBAC), *Contemporary Nurse*, 34 (1): 77–84.

Redshaw, M., Hennegan, J. and Kruske, S. (2014) Holding the baby: early mother–infant contact after childbirth and outcomes, *Midwifery*, 30 (5): 177–87.

Regan, J., Thompson, A. and DeFranco, E. (2013) The influence of mode of delivery on breastfeeding initiation in women with a prior caesarean delivery: a population based study, *Breastfeeding Medicine*, 8 (2): 181–6.

Renner, R.M., Eden, K.B., Osterweil, B.S., Chan, B.K. and Guise, J.M. (2007) Informational factors influencing patients' childbirth preferences after prior caesarean, *American Journal of Obstetrics and Gynecology*, 196 (5): e14–16.

Royal College of Obstetricians and Gynaecologists (RCOG) (2015) *Birth After Previous Caesarean Birth*, Green-top Guideline GTG45. London: RCOG [https://www.rcog.org.uk/en/guidelines-research-services/guidelines/gtg45/; accessed 25 November 2015].

Rozen, G., Ugoni, A. and Sheehan, P.M. (2011) A new perspective on VBAC: a retrospective cohort study, *Women and Birth*, 24 (1): 3–9.

Scaffadi, R.M., Posmontier, B., Bloch, J.R. and Wittmann-Price, R. (2014) The relationship between personal knowledge and decision self-efficacy in choosing trial of labor after caesarean, *Journal of Midwifery and Women's Health*, 59 (3): 246–53.

Schoorel, E.N.C., van Kuijk, S.M.J., Melman, S., Nijhuis, J.G., Smits, L.J.M., Aardenburg, R. et al. (2013) Vaginal birth after a caesarean section: the development of a Western European population-based prediction model for deliveries at term, *BJOG: An International Journal of Obstetrics and Gynaecology*, 121 (2): 194–201.

Scioscia, M., Vimercati, A., Cito, L., Chironna, E., Scattarella, D. and Selvaggi, L.E. (2008) Social determinants of the increasing caesarean section rate in Italy, *Minerva Ginecologica*, 60 (2): 115–20.

Shorten, A., Shorten, B. and Kennedy, H.P. (2014) Complexities of choice after prior cesarean: a narrative analysis, *Birth*, 41 (2): 178–84.

Shorten, A., Shorten, B., Keogh, J., West, S. and Morris, J. (2005) Making choices for childbirth: a randomized controlled trial of a decision-aid for informed birth after caesarean, *Birth*, 32 (4): 252–61.

Villar, J., Carroli, G., Zavaleta, N., Donner, A., Wojdyla, D., Faundes, A. et al. (2007) Maternal and neonatal individual risks and benefits associated with caesarean delivery: multi-centre prospective study, *British Medical Journal*, 335 (7628): 1025.

Weaver, J. (2000) Talking about caesarean section, *MIDIRS Midwifery Digest*, 10 (4): 487–90.

Whitelaw, N., Bhattacharya, S., McLernon, D. and Black, M. (2014) Internet information on birth options after caesarean compared to the RCOG leaflet: a web survey, *BMC Pregnancy and Childbirth*, 14: 361.

Zanardo, V., Svegliado, G., Cavallin, F., Guistardi, A., Cosmi, E., Litta, P. et al. (2010) Elective cesarean delivery: does it have a negative effect on breastfeeding?, *Birth*, 37 (4): 275–9.

11

When labour slows or stops

Karen Jackson

Introduction

Slow progress in the first stage of labour may have major implications for women's experience of childbirth. Yet its definition seems to be absent or arbitrary in many of the articles written on this topic. Therefore, the management of slow progress is not based on any form of solid evidence base. Women have been and continue to be subjected to high levels of technological interventions, when labour is considered to be 'slow' or to have stopped. There are known adverse consequences of the interventions themselves.

This chapter looks at what slow progress is and why it is important, time constraints in labour, progress in labour and the development and subsequent widespread use of the partogram, the normal parameters of labour, the medical management of slow progress and how progress of labour can be assessed, including less invasive methods than vaginal examination. It will also examine approaches to childbirth when labour slows or stops and present cases based on real experiences where water immersion and other strategies have been used.

Slow progress of labour and why is it important

There is no consensus on what constitutes 'slow progress' of labour; it appears to be an arbitrary assessment of when progress does not follow the prescribed normal parameters. Bugg et al. (2013) concur with this, stating that the definition of slow progress remains controversial. Within various studies, slow progress of labour seems to be a vague and ill-defined phenomenon, with little agreement on the diagnostic criteria for 'dystocia' (Kjærgaard et al., 2009). Maternal characteristics that are associated with slow progress of labour are maternal age above 35 years, primiparity, obesity and a short maternal stature of less than 150 cm (Greenberg et al., 2007; Shields et al., 2007; Lowe and Corwin, 2011). Fetal reasons include: malpositions, non-engagement of fetal head and cephalo-pelvic disproportion (Simkin and Ancheta, 2011). Simkin and Ancheta (2011) also suggest non-biological reasons for slow progress such as emotional dystocia and iatrogenic dystocia.

There are numerous terminologies for slow progress of labour. Prolonged labour, labour dystocia, uterine inertia, failure to progress, delay in first/second stage of labour and dysfunctional labour are just a few examples, but what is striking is the explicit negativity of the terminologies, implying that women's bodies have not performed efficiently enough and have been defective in the child-bearing process. Cluett et al. (2004) suggest 'slower than expected labour', which provides an antidote to the typically unconstructive language often used in obstetrics. Prolonged or slow progress of labour is one of the major reasons for caesarean sections (20% of caesareans in the UK, over 50% in the USA) and instrumental deliveries, and was thought to be responsible for an increase in maternal and fetal morbidity, but by and large the nature of these morbidities were not expanded on in many of the articles reviewed for this chapter (Hall, 2001; Cluett et al., 2004; Bugg et al., 2013). El-Sayed (2012) suggests a higher rate of caesarean section and chorioamnionitis for the mother, and higher admission to intensive care for the neonate related to a labour lasting over 30 hours. Kjærgaard et al. (2009) question whether the increased morbidity is actually associated with 'slow labour' or whether it is an iatrogenic consequence of the interventions themselves in these labours.

Little in the way of good quality evidence exists to assess what exactly prolonged labour is, if it is always pathological or if it can be a variation in physiology, and if it does always have an adverse effect on birth outcomes. The paradox of a biomedical management of slow progress – with its use of oxytocics and/or artificial rupture of membranes leading to increased use of epidurals, resulting in more instrumental deliveries, and causing maternal and fetal morbidity – appears to be conveniently ignored (Kabiru et al., 2001; Patel and Murphy, 2004; O'Mahony et al., 2010). In addition, intervention in labour is also associated with lower satisfaction with the overall childbearing experience (Glazener et al., 1995; Green et al., 1998, 2003; Baston et al., 2008).

Time constraints in labour

Applying time constraints to labour has been a familiar part of maternity care for at least half a century. This coincided with the move from childbearing women giving birth at home to giving birth in increasingly larger maternity units (Walsh, 2010). In contemporary obstetrics, where the vast majority of women give birth in a hospital setting, there exists a cynical view that time limits had more to do with managing busy labour suites in an institutionalized, assembly-line business-like fashion (Perkins, 2004), rather than (or at least concurrent with) concern for mothers' and babies' welfare.

As discussed, slow progress is manifestly connected with higher levels of interventions in labour and ultimately a major reason for caesarean section (Bugg et al., 2013). However, the phenomenon of slow progress of labour and the reasons behind it have been hotly contested in recent years. Indeed, the very notion of what constitutes 'normal' progress during labour remains controversial. In 1969, O'Driscoll, famous for popularizing active management of labour, advised that any nulliparous woman with a cervical dilatation rate of less than 1 cm an hour required treatment, as this constituted 'slow progress' (O'Driscoll et al., 1969). He aimed for all nulliparous women to be 'delivered' within 12 hours of active labour. The only component of the active management regime that has subsequently been shown to be effective in reducing length of labour is one-to one continuous support (Walsh 2010). Latterly, a rate of 0.5 cm an hour (Albers, 1999; Cesario, 2004) is the accepted rate of progress. If progress falls below this rate, treatment should be considered according to NICE guidance (2008).

Progress in labour and the development of the partogram

Once labour has established, it is considered normal practice to carefully moni-tor the progress of labour to ensure that it does not detract from a normal path-way. In 1954, Friedman proposed a graph, known as the Friedman curve, to assess normal progress in terms of length of labour. This graph was based on observations of cervical dilatation, and descent of the fetal head, plotted in rela-tion to time in hours from the onset of labour. The result was a typical S-shaped curve that showed the duration of normal labour with healthy outcomes for mothers and babies (Friedman, 1954; Cesario, 2004). Figure 11.1 shows the plot-ted curves arising from the research of various researchers. Friedman's research has been criticized for not being rigorous and representative, as the original sample inappropriately included 'non low risk' nulliparous labouring women (Neal et al., 2010).

This early partogram or cervicogram was subsequently used to plot a rate of expected cervical dilation of approximately 1 cm an hour. The partogram became an integral aspect of labour 'management' in many industrialized countries for at

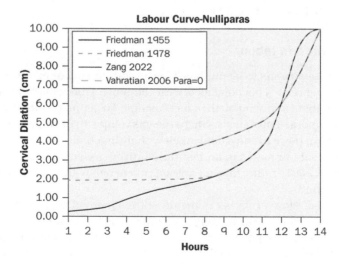

Figure 11.1 Friedman's curve.

Source: Adapted from Joy and Peng (2011).

least the rest of the last century, with little questioning of its provenance or value. In 1972, Philpott and Castle added alert, transfer and action lines. These were developed in the context of a developing country, namely Rhodesia, where obstructed or prolonged labour in a remote rural location could have catastrophic effects for mother and fetus.

The widespread use of partograms for monitoring progress of labour has been the subject of a recent systematic review. Lavendar et al. (2013) examined outcomes for women and babies comparing partogram use with no partogram. They found no evidence to support the routine use of the partogram in women who commenced labour spontaneously at term.

Normal parameters of labour

The latent phase of labour can be extremely challenging for women and their lived experiences of latency. The importance of recognizing when women are in the active phase of labour to reduce unnecessary intervention is well documented (Cheyne et al., 2006; Spiby et al., 2008). An entire chapter of this book is devoted to the latent phase of labour (see Chapter 6) and it will not be discussed in any depth here. However, in a large, multicentre, prospective observational study, based on data from 26,838 labours, Zhang et al. (2010) concluded that multiparas may not enter 'active' labour until cervical dilatation of at least 5 cm. For nulliparas, active labour may commence even later. Current 'diagnosis' of active labour in the UK is stated as cervical dilatation of 4 cm or more (NICE, 2014). The American College of Obstetricians and Gynaecologists (ACOG, 2013) have attempted to stem the rising caesarean section rate by recommending that active labour not be considered until the cervix is at least 6 cm dilated.

In 1999, Albers challenged the cervical dilatation of 1 cm an hour rule. She found that length of active normal labours in a low-risk population of women in nine different centres in the USA had an upper normal parameter of 17.5 hours (versus Friedman's 8.5 hours) in primgravid women and 13.8 hours (versus Friedman's 7 hours) for multiparous women, with no statistically significant differences in outcomes.

NICE (2014) pooled findings from descriptive studies and reported that the range of upper limits of length of labour for primigravid women was 8.2–19.4 hours and for multigravid women 12.5–14.9 hours. However, NICE do stipulate that these findings are flawed due to standard deviations being used on the assumption that normal labour has a normal distribution, which is not the case.

Since 2000, others have questioned Friedman's rigid parameters for normal labour (Zhang et al., 2002; Cesario, 2004). In their systematic review of 25 studies, Neal et al. (2010) found that nulliparous women, whose labours had commenced spontaneously, had slower than expected cervical dilatation rates and thus longer active labours than would have been traditionally anticipated. They concluded that a 'fast' estimated cervical dilatation rate of 1 cm an hour is likely to result in an over-diagnosis of labour dystocia and the consequent overuse of interventions to augment labour. ACOG (2013) have also stated that contemporary labour may progress substantially slower than has been thought historically.

Medical management of 'slow progress' of labour

In contemporary obstetric practice, if a labour does not follow the defined pattern of progress, then intervention will ensue to correct 'dystocia' or 'prolonged' labour, commencing what Inch (1985) would describe as a 'cascade of intervention'. In this instance, the cascade is likely to the prescribing of a syntocinon infusion and/or artificial rupture of membranes, followed by epidural, leading to a known increased risk of an assisted birth (Liu and Sia, 2004). Although syntocinon is used widely to augment labour, it has some potentially serious side effects, including hyper-stimulation of the uterus leading to ruptured uterus, and increased risk of morbidity and mortality for mother and/or baby (NICE, 2008). Bugg et al. (2013) reviewed eight studies involving 1338 low-risk labouring women. Their purpose was to explore the belief that oxytocin use reduces the rate of caesarean section in cases of slow progress in the first stage of labour. They found no differences in caesarean section rates when intravenous oxytocin administration was compared with an expectant management of slow progress of labour. There was a reduction of 2 hours in the labour length under the oxytocic regimen, but this was not associated with any differences in maternal or neonatal wellbeing. Furthermore, artificial rupture of membranes does not significantly reduce length of labour, but may increase the risk of a caesarean section, according to Smyth et al. (2013).

Reed (2011) states that any form of augmentation must alter the physiology of labour, thus interfering in the natural interaction of hormones. These findings suggest that the decision to use oxytocics to augment labour should be a considered one, especially in an essentially normal labour that happens not to conform to a medically dictated timeframe (NICE, 2008; Martin, 2009; Reed, 2011; Smyth et al., 2013).

In a minority of women, augmentation is absolutely the correct course of action; for an even smaller number of women, true disproportion between size of the fetus and size of the woman's pelvis does arise and a caesarean section may be the only possible mode of birth (Bugg et al., 2013). Obstetricians and midwives must be vigilant in these cases that are genuinely deviating from normal.

Assessing progress of labour

A common method of assessing progress of labour is by vaginal examination. This has become a routine procedure in labour care, with little research evidence to support its value. Reed (2011) emphasizes the limited usefulness of vaginal examinations, as they only provide a 'snapshot' of what the cervix is doing at a particular moment. They cannot provide information on the state of the cervix previously, or the state of the cervix in the future. Vaginal examination is a highly invasive procedure, and can increase the risk of introducing infection (Shepherd et al., 2010). In women who have survived sexual abuse, women with 'female genital mutilation' and women who are anxious, vaginal examination can be an extremely distressing (sometimes impossible) procedure. Crowther et al. (2000) describe vaginal examinations as not always reliable, invasive, subjective and of unproven benefit. Walsh (2011) questions the confidence practitioners have in the findings of vaginal examinations, as inter-observer reliability of the procedure is notoriously poor (Clement, 1994). Despite this, the NICE intrapartum guidelines (2014) state that women in established first stage of labour should be offered a vaginal examination four hourly, and in the second stage, one should be offered every hour. This does not seem to be consistent with available evidence.

Experienced midwives recount a number of alternatives to vaginal examination for assessing progress of labour. These include abdominal palpation, 'the purple line', Rhombus of Michaelis, and the general behaviour and sounds made by women during different rhythms of labour (Walsh, 2010). However, very limited research has been conducted on these practices.

Stuart (2000) describes palpating the abdomen every 2–3 hours to assess progress, monitoring descent of the presenting part through the birth canal. In good midwifery practice, abdominal palpation is required before vaginal examination so as to collate the information from the two examinations and improve accuracy of the findings (Jay and Hamilton, 2008). Using abdominal palpation alone to assess progress of labour does not seem to have been effectively researched.

Hobbs (1998) described visualization of the 'purple line' that appears from the women's anal margin, which gradually extends to the nape of the buttocks. The extension of the purple line is directly related to the stage of labour. Once the nape of the buttocks is reached, the woman's cervix will be fully dilated. In their longitudinal study of 144 labouring women, Shepherd et al. (2010) found that the purple line was present in 76% of the sample and that there was a medium positive correlation between length of the purple line and cervical dilation. They conclude that the purple line, when present, could be used to assess progress in labour, although they do state that further research is required. It is worth noting that the line may not always be 'purple'; it may be red or appear dark in some women depending on skin colour (RCM, 2012a).

The Rhombus of Michaelis is a kite-shaped area located above the ligaments connecting the sacrum to the ilea and which becomes more flexible during labour. The shape is formed when the descending fetal head pushes the sacrum and coccyx backwards and is most visible during the early second stage of labour (Wickham and Sutton, 2005). The Rhombus of Michaelis is well reported anecdotally (Wickham and Sutton, 2005), but women have to be in a standing or all-fours position for it to be visible, and again using this phenomenon to assess progress of labour has not been reliably evaluated.

Practice point

If you have not used these methods to assess progress of labour before, when you next care for a childbearing woman in labour, observe for the purple line and/or the Rhombus of Michaelis in conjunction with your usual practice of assessing labour progress. This will enhance your experience and confidence in these methods.

The changing behaviour of women during labour is well recognized anecdotally, but again little research has been conducted in this area. The characteristics of contractions have been studied by Stuart (2000), basically describing contractions changing from relatively painless and irregular in the early part of labour, to strong, frequent (4–5 in 10 minutes) expulsive contractions, often with an accompanying urge to push in the latter stage of labour. Burvill (2002) found that breathing patterns changed throughout labour from normal to exaggerated panicked breathing, to deep controlled breathing to grunting throat sounds. She also found that conversation continued normally in early labour, with women becoming increasingly withdrawn and quiet in the later stages of labour. Burvill (2002) also looked at movement and posture and found that women move during contractions initially, before tending to bend forward and grasp the abdomen. Later in the labour their movement becomes more focused; they may stay in one area/space and sway the hips during contractions, or they may also wish to hold onto something during a contraction (see Table 11.1).

Dixon and Foureur (2010) state that vaginal examinations can arguably be considered both an intervention and an essential clinical assessment tool. They recommend that vaginal examinations should be used judiciously when there is a need for more information and it cannot be obtained from external observation of the woman in labour.

Clearly, there is a need in some cases to conduct a vaginal examination in labour, but this should not become the standard approach to care for all women (Dixon and Foureur, 2010). There is a need for all midwifery skills, including non-invasive methods of assessing progress in labour. More research is needed in this area (Stuart, 2000; Burvill, 2002; Chapman, 2003; Dixon and Foureur, 2010).

Midwifery approaches when labour progress stops or slows

Midwives can no doubt recount numerous occasions when a woman's contractions in the full throng of labour appeared either to stop or slow down. This phenomenon is well recognized by independent/experienced home birth midwives who are entirely comfortable with this kind of 'plateau'. They see this cessation of contractions as a part of the normal rhythm of labour, and not to be considered problematic if mother and baby are well (Duff, 2005). Indeed, Gaskin (2003) was taught the concept of 'Pasmo' by a Puerto Rican nurse in 2003. It means the stopping or even going backwards of a labour that has established, with an accompanying reduction in cervical dilatation. It is seen as physiological in Puerto Rican culture and these labours re-establish in time, with no apparent problems for mother or baby. It may be viewed as part of the finely tuned balance between labour hormones or the 'dance' of labour as it is sometimes referred to.

In the context of the labour suite, where the 'clock is ticking', what action the midwife takes if labour progress stops or slows could potentially decide between maintaining an unusual but still normal pathway to a straightforward birth, or immediately alerting the medical team. The latter will establish a more technological approach to the labour and may well lead to the ubiquitously documented

Table 11.1 Assessing progress of labour.

Cervical dilatation and women's behaviour and noises during labour

Criteria	0–3	3–4	4–7	7–9	9–10
Contractions: increasing in length, frequency and strength (Stuart, 2000)	Tight uterus with painless contractions. Sometimes irregular and may stop	2 in 10 minutes; increasingly regular and lasting 20–40 seconds	3 in 10 minutes; regular usually with bearable pain, lasting around 60 seconds	3 or 4 in 10 minutes; regular with increasing pain	4 or 5 in 10 minutes; regular and at their most painful. May experience an increasing urge to push
Breathing and conversation (Burvill, 2002)	No change	May have exaggerated panic-like breathing; may become chatty	Deeper breathing like a sigh, controlled pronounced start of voice breathing; speaks less	Becomes focused. The woman becomes quiet and conversation stops. Focused on breathing, which slows down with contraction. Makes grunting throat sounds, cries out with expiration	
Movement and posture (Burvill, 2002)	Moves during contraction		Grasps abdomen and bends forward	Holds on to something during a contraction. Sways hips during contraction, very focused, concentrated movements. Less mobile overall	

Source: Adapted from Chapman (2003).

'cascade of intervention'. The commencement of synthetic oxytocics to augment labour is quite likely. Labours augmented with syntocinon commonly lead to increased epidural use (Anim-Somuah et al., 2011). Anim-Somuah et al. (2011) conducted a systematic review of epidural use in labour. They found that there was a statistically significant difference in instrumental birth in women who used epidurals compared with those who did not. There were no differences in maternal satisfaction with pain relief. Increased morbidity in terms of trauma for mother and baby are well recognized in instrumental births (Kabiru et al., 2001; Patel and Murphy, 2004; O'Mahony et al., 2010).

Supportive strategies when labour slows or stops include: maintaining a positive attitude and a belief in the woman's ability to give birth (Davies, 2011), resting, changing position and posture, touch, emotional support, providing food and drink, and application of hot towels to the lower back (Simkin and Ancheta, 2011). These strategies appear to be pragmatic and based on experience and common sense. But they are also anecdotal and while midwives will undoubtedly intuitively 'know' that these strategies are likely to help, they do not have any 'scientific' credence and are thus not based on so-called 'authoritative knowledge' in the current evidence-based culture in which midwives practise. A body of evidence is now beginning to emerge demonstrating the positive effects of less technological and more normalized and humanistic approaches to slow labour.

Water immersion

The physiological benefits of water immersion are well documented (Figure 11.2). Water immersion leads to buoyancy, which increases mobility and movement, which in turn can facilitate neuro-hormonal changes in labour thus alleviating pain, increasing uterine perfusion, reducing labour duration, decreasing the need

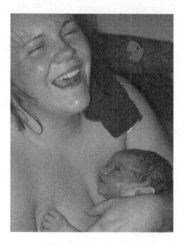

Figure 11.2 Water immersion in labour.

Source: Copyright free.

for intervention, encouraging optimal fetal positioning and potentially optimizing physiological processes and progress of labour (Aird et al., 1997; Ginesi, 1998a, 1998b; Garland and Jones, 2000; Otigbah et al., 2000; Moneta et al., 2001; Geissbuehler et al., 2004; Cluett and Burns, 2009). However, the use of water immersion when labour slows or stops or is diagnosed as 'dystocia' is less well explored.

Cluett et al. (2004) conducted a randomized controlled trial comparing 48 nulliparous women labouring in water and 48 nulliparous women who received standard management of 'dystocia' in first stage of labour. This management consisted of amniotomy if membranes were intact, followed by commencement of syntocinon infusion after 2 hours. Women in the water immersion group reported less pain and increased satisfaction, and had less need for epidural analgesia. They also had fewer obstetric interventions. The researchers concluded that this was another management option for slow progress of labour.

Two further studies comparing immersion in water with land labour found that those immersed in water had significantly reduced duration of labour (Zanetti-Dallenback et al., 2007; Thoni et al., 2010). Cluett and Burns' (2009) systematic review of 12 trials (3243 women) also found a reduction in the duration of the first stage of labour, in addition to a significant reduction in epidural and spinal use in women who used water immersion during labour. However, some studies have not reported the same positive effects on labour; for example, Eriksson et al. (1997) did not observe a reduction in the length of labour. It is thought that this might be due to the women entering the pool earlier in labour in the two studies in which there was a reduction, whereas in the latter study, women immersed in water when labour was well established.

Case 11.1: Tamara

Tamara was a 23-year-old student nurse who was pregnant with her first child. At 39 weeks gestation she commenced spontaneous labour. Tamara was extremely keen to achieve a normal labour and birth, and remained mobile and upright throughout her labour. Labour progressed extremely slowly. After 18 hours of being in labour, her contractions started to space out to about one every 10 minutes. The midwife in attendance was monitoring maternal and fetal wellbeing and all was well. After another hour, Tamara requested a vaginal examination. The midwife found that the cervix was fully dilated and the fetal head was about 1 cm below the ischial spines.

Tamara was exhausted but still determined to avoid any intervention during her labour. Tamara immersed in water for a while, used the birthing ball, and received lavender aromatherapy massage. The contractions returned slightly more regularly: 2 in 10 minutes. She stated that she did not want any pharmacological pain relief even though she was becoming quite distressed. Two hours later, she felt the urge to push. Tamara proceeded to push using her own physiological urges. Again progress was slow. After pushing in many different positions – on the toilet, on a birthing stool, left lateral – the fetal head was barely visible.

Tamara realized that she needed some help and agreed to be seen by the obstetric registrar. The baby was delivered using rotational Keillands forceps; once the head had been slightly rotated, her baby was delivered with relative ease. Mother and baby were in good condition. Far from being disappointed, Tamara was delighted with her birth experience, as she felt she had been listened to and had remained in control and part of the decision-making process throughout. She felt that she had given normal birth her 'best shot'.

Practice point

The coordinating midwife was keen to call the obstetric registrar much earlier in Tamara's labour. What would you do in your own practice faced with this scenario?

Continuous support in labour

The benefits of the continuous presence of a supportive companion during labour and birth are widely known. In 1991, Kennell and colleagues published the results of a trial conducted in a modern hospital in the USA, in which they randomly assigned 212 women to continuous support with a doula, 200 women to a female 'observer'-only group and 204 to a control group who received usual care. They found that the continuous support group, and to a lesser extent the observed group, were significantly different to the control group in relation to reduced numbers of caesarean sections, instrumental deliveries, less use of oxytocin and shorter labours. The researchers called for a review of obstetric practices based on the dramatic differences found when women received this continuous social support.

More recently, in a Cochrane systematic review of 22 trials involving 15,288 women, Hodnett et al. (2013) found that those who received continuous support in labour were more likely to have a spontaneous vaginal birth, less likely to have intrapartum analgesia including epidurals and less likely to report dissatisfaction. In addition, their labours were shorter, they were less likely to have a caesarean or an instrumental vaginal birth, and babies were less likely to have a low Apgar score at 5 minutes.

Hodnett et al. (2013) suggested theoretical explanations for the positive effects of labour support on childbirth outcomes. They hypothesized that labour support enhances labour physiology and mothers' feelings of control and competence, reducing reliance on technology and medical interventions. Birth companions are likely to support women in their choices of upright positions, provide information, emotional support and advice, act as advocates and enhance comfort measures. These actions reduce anxiety, thus moderating the stressors of childbirth.

> **Practice point**
>
> Supporting women in longer labours is acceptable providing that there are no issues with maternal and/or fetal condition. Any deviation from normal should be referred to an appropriate health practitioner (NMC, 2012). If in any doubt, it is advisable to seek a second opinion.

Massage

Massage has been acknowledged throughout history for its health benefits. The use of massage to reduce pain has been well researched and reviewed (Field, 2010; Smith et al., 2012; Gallo et al., 2013). The physical contact required of massage potentiates relaxation by reducing stress. The physiological processes are thought to be due to a reduction in cortisol and norepinephrine (Chang et al., 2002; Field, 2010), an increase in serotonin and stimulation of endorphin release. This subsequently improves oxygen perfusion and toxin excretion through the lymphatic system (Zwelling et al., 2006). And there is a growing body of evidence demonstrating that massage has considerable benefits not just for reducing pain, but also for reducing the duration of labour.

Field et al. (1997) found that 28 labouring women who received head, shoulder, back, hand and foot massage for 20 minutes every hour for 5 hours reported less stress, reduced pain but also significantly shorter labours and time in hospital than women who did not receive massage. Simkin and O'Hara (2002) reviewed two trials that appeared to indicate that massage relieves pain, reduces anxiety and enhances the progress of labour, with no identified risks – although the authors did state that more scientific research is needed to provide clearer conclusions. In a randomized controlled trial conducted by Khoda Karami et al. (2007), 60 labouring women received Swedish massage to sacrum, buttocks, shoulders, waist, feet and hands during different phases of labour. The women in the experimental group experienced a significantly shorter first stage of labour than those in the control group.

> **Case 11.2: Fatima**
>
> Fatima was a 28-year-old primigravida, 39 + 5 weeks pregnant. She had been in established labour for 8 hours. Two of her sisters were present with her during the labour, as she did not think that her husband was the best person to help her at this time. Her contractions were very strong and intense and she was progressing well. She was upright and mobilizing in the birthing room, leaning over one of her sisters during a strong contraction. Gradually, her contractions became further apart, until they virtually stopped. There were no concerns regarding maternal or fetal condition. It was suggested that she try water immersion but Fatima declined. She went for a walk outside of the labour suite, but

when she returned her contractions were still absent. She became quite distressed through sheer frustration. Her sisters consoled her, and started to intuitively massage her shoulders, her abdomen, back and hips. She found this very relaxing, and after 10 minutes her contractions returned, becoming intense and strong, 3 every 10 minutes. Her sisters continued to massage Fatima for the remainder of her labour, and two hours later she gave birth to a healthy baby boy, in a standing position.

Reflection point

In your own practice, what would give you the confidence to support a woman in this situation when labour stops or slows?

Upright positions and mobilization

Throughout history, women have naturally adopted upright positions for labour and birth. Upright positions are commonly accepted as including sitting upright, kneeling, squatting, standing and being on all fours. Gradually, however, during the twentieth century, for socio-cultural reasons and apparent convenience of the accoucheur (ease of performing vaginal examinations, monitoring fetal heart rate, etc.), women – mainly in high-income countries – have tended to labour in a semi-recumbent position, generally on a bed (Gholitabar, 2009).

There are numerous theoretical advantages to upright positions in labour: gravity can help with progress, there is a reduced risk of aorto-caval compression, the fetus is better positioned in the uterus leading to more efficient contractions and increased pelvic outlet when in a squatting or kneeling position (MIDIRS, 2008).

In 2002, Simkin and O'Hara undertook a systematic review of non-pharmacologic relief of pain during labour. They looked at 14 studies of movement and positioning in labour and concluded that for low-risk women adopting a predominantly upright position during labour, in addition to relieving pain, it may speed up labour and increase maternal comfort. In their systematic review of 21 studies involving 3706 women, Lawrence et al. (2009) found that walking and adopting upright positions in labour reduced labour by approximately one hour. There were no apparent increases in the need for intervention or any negative impact on maternal or fetal/neonatal wellbeing. Kamud et al. (2013) randomized 60 mainly nulliparous women into upright positions and usual care during active labour. The women who had adopted upright positions during active labour had on average a two-hour shorter labour. Their contractions were more intense when upright, but women in this group also reported being more comfortable in the upright position. No differences in maternal or fetal/neonatal wellbeing were observed.

Eating and drinking in labour

Until relatively recently, restricting the intake of food and drink for childbearing women during labour was routinely practised in many countries (Singata et al., 2010). This was due to a theoretical risk of acidic gastric aspiration, and subsequent Mendelson's syndrome should general anaesthesia be required (Mendelson, 1946). Fasting during labour cannot guarantee an empty stomach or a high pH should an operative delivery become necessary (RCM, 2012b). Mild ketosis during labour may be considered to be a normal physiological state (RCM, 2012b). However, according to Foulkes and Dumoulin (1985) and Broach and Newton (1988), if ketosis, starvation and fatigue occur in combination, inefficient uterine action, increased active management and a subsequent increase in instrumental delivery may ensue.

Dehydration in particular has been postulated as a possible cause of slow progress in labour (Simkin and Ancheta, 2011). But studies have focused on the medical treatment of intravenous therapy for the treatment of slow progress (Garite et al., 2000), which does not resonate with the normalized, woman-centred ethos of this book.

In a randomized controlled trial, O'Sullivan et al. (2009) found that consumption of a light diet during labour did not influence obstetric or neonatal outcomes in 2426 participants, nor did it increase the incidence of vomiting. Women who are allowed to eat in labour have similar lengths of labour and operative delivery rates to those allowed water only.

Eating and drinking in labour enables women to feel normal and healthy, maintains their energy levels and helps to mediate against exhaustion. It also has many psychological benefits, such as providing reassurance and comfort, whereas withholding food and drink is seen as authoritarian, intimidating and can increase feelings of apprehension (RCM, 2012b). Singata et al. (2010) and NICE (2014) both recommend that low-risk women should be able to eat a light diet and drink in labour.

Aromatherapy

Little evidence exists on the effectiveness of aromatherapy for labour, but as it gains popularity with childbearing women, it is likely that more research will be conducted to support its use.

Zahra and Leila (2013) conducted a randomized controlled trial (RCT) in Iran with women randomly assigned to either massage only or aromatherapy massage with lavender oil. Intensity of pain was significantly lower in the aromatherapy massage group and both first and second stages of labour were shorter. It should be noted, however, that only 30 women were assigned to each group in this study.

In 1999, Burns and colleagues conducted an evaluative study of the use of aromatherapy in intrapartum care. The study included a sample of 8058 mothers across the risk spectrum between 1990 and 1998. The findings demonstrated that aromatherapy alleviated anxiety and fear, as well as appearing to reduce the need for additional pain relief, thus resulting in a lower than average epidural rate (Burns et al., 1999). Then in 2007, Burns et al. undertook a pilot RCT to demonstrate the feasibility of undertaking a comprehensive trial on the effects of aromatherapy in labour; there were no associated adverse effects on either maternal or neonatal outcomes when using the essential oils in the trial. And in a study of 1079 labouring women, Dhany et al. (2012) assessed the outcomes of an aromatherapy and massage service and found that it reduced all types of intrapartum anaesthesia.

It should be acknowledged that aromatherapy is often used in conjunction with massage and/or water immersion.

Case 11.3: Alana

Alana was 32 years old, 39 weeks pregnant, and a gravida 3 para 2. Her labour had commenced spontaneously, and she had been in established labour for around 6 hours. Her husband was present but did not engage much in what was happening. An hour earlier, a vaginal examination had been requested by Alana and her cervix was found to be 5 cm, with the fetal head 2 cm below the ischial spines; the membranes were still intact. Alana's contractions had been frequent and strong (3–4 in 10 minutes), she was upright and mobile and had stated she wanted her labour to be as natural as possible. Her contractions initially spread to 2 in ten minutes, then 1 in ten. There was no immediate concern, as mother and fetus were both well. However, Alana was becoming quite frustrated as she felt that her labour had ceased.

Alana was advised to go for a walk, use the birthing ball and take advantage of some aromatherapy and possibly the pool. Alana went for a walk with her husband, and she also tried the birthing ball but did not find it comfortable. After about an hour and after some discussion, Alana said she would like to try the birthing pool, with some added aromatherapy. The birthing pool was subsequently prepared and drops of clarysage, lavender and jasmine were added. On entering the pool, Alana immediately said that she found it very relaxing. Her contractions quickly returned, strong at 4 in ten minutes, and although Alana had initially said she did not want to give birth in the pool, once in, she changed her mind and within 20 minutes gave birth to a healthy baby girl.

Reflection point

If you do not use aromatherapy oils in your maternity units, what could you do to address this?

Acupuncture and acupressure

The use of acupuncture during labour has been found to reduce mean pain scores, and result in less pharmacological pain relief and augmentation (Skilnand et al., 2002). In another randomized controlled trial, acupressure demonstrated reduced pain scores and length of labour (Lee et al., 2004). There is a dearth of good quality evidence exploring the use of acupuncture and acupressure in childbirth, although there is promise in using these complementary therapies as an alternative to augmenting labour via a medicalized route.

Key points: suggestions for supporting women when labour has slowed or stopped

- Midwives can join Trust guidelines groups in an effort to ensure that evidence-based guidelines are developed that recognize the many factors affecting labour length in normal childbirth. Alternatively, ask for draft guidelines to be circulated and give constructive feedback supported by good quality research/evidence.
- Women's informed choices should be respected, even if they do not conform to medical advice (NMC, 2015).
- Midwives must always assess the clinical picture competently, including maternal and fetal wellbeing. If there are specific concerns, then medical intervention may be appropriate.
- Where appropriate, midwives should always act as advocates for women to protect them from any unwanted or unnecessary intervention (NMC, 2015).
- If aromatherapy is not available in your Trust, be proactive in visiting Trusts where aromatherapy is routinely used (see contact details at the end of this chapter). Seek advice on how this service was started. Support from midwife managers/leaders is vital. Put together an evidence-based proposal for setting up an aromatherapy service. A commitment to education and training for all midwives is essential. Introduce education and training in the use of aromatherapy into student midwives' curriculum.
- If you are challenged regarding your care of women during a labour that has slowed or stopped, you need to be able to justify your position. The woman making an informed choice not to receive an intervention is an excellent rationale. Also ensure that you can cite good quality research/evidence to support your actions.

Conclusion

This chapter has explored what slow progress of labour is and why it is important, time constraints in labour, progress in labour and the development of the partogram, the normal parameters of labour, medical management of 'slow progress' of labour, assessing progress in labour, and midwifery approaches when labour progress stops or slows, including water immersion, one-to-one support and aromatherapy.

The clinical imperative to speed up normal labour because it makes it more efficient or fit more neatly into the organizational needs of a busy labour suite has been challenged. It is hoped that the evidence together with what midwives already instinctively know, will change the technocratic approach to labour and safeguard a physiological labour (or as physiological as possible), even when it may have stopped or be 'slower than expected'.

Further reading

Davies, S. (2011) A longer labour and birth . . . one size does not fit all, in S. Donna (ed.) *Promoting Normal Birth: Research, reflections and guidelines.* Chester-le-Street: Fresh Heart Publishing. An evidence-based overview of 'longer labours', including a more advanced understanding of the physiology of labour, and practical approaches when a labour appears long.

Simkin, P. and Ancheta, R. (2011) *The Labor Progress Handbook: Early interventions to prevent and treat dystocia* (3rd edn). Chichester: Wiley-Blackwell. A book devoted entirely to the topic of labour 'dystocia'. It provides excellent anecdotal and evidence-based hints and tips for supporting women through longer labours

Walsh, D. (2010) Labour rhythms, in D. Walsh and S. Downe (eds) *Essential Midwifery Practice: Intrapartum care.* Chichester: Wiley-Blackwell. A thorough, academic yet accessible discussion of all aspects of labour, including 'rhythms' in mid-labour.

Useful contact

Contact details regarding maternity aromatherapy service: Ellaine Allright, Lead Midwife for Aromatherapy, Nottingham University Hospitals NHS Trust [Ellaine.allright@nuh.nhs.uk].

References

Aird, A., Luckas, M., Buckett, W. and Bousfielf, P. (1997) Effects of intrapartum hydrotherapy on labour parameters, *Australian and New Zealand Journal of Obstetrics and Gynaecology*, 37 (2): 137–42.

Albers, L. (1999) The duration of labour in healthy women, *Journal of Perinatology*, 19 (2): 114–19.

American College of Obstetricians and Gynaecologists (ACOG) (2013) Obstetric care consensus no. 1: safe prevention of the primary cesarean delivery, *Obstetrics and Gynaecology*, 123 (3): 693–711.

Anim-Somuah, M., Smyth, R.M.D. and Jones, L. (2011) Epidural versus non-epidural or no analgesia in labour, *Cochrane Database of Systematic Reviews*, 12: CD000331.

Baston, H., Rijnders, M., Green, J. and Buitendijk, S. (2008) Looking back on birth three years later: factors associated with a negative appraisal in England and in the Netherlands, *Journal of Reproductive and Infant Psychology*, 26 (4): 323–39.

Broach, J. and Newton, N. (1988) Food and beverages in labour. Part II: The effects of cessation of oral intake during labour, *Birth*, 15 (2): 88–92.

Bugg, G., Siddiqui, F. and Thornton, J. (2013) Oxytocin versus no treatment or delayed treatment for slow progress in the first stage of spontaneous labour, *Cochrane Database of Systematic Reviews*, 6: CD007123.

Burns, E., Blamey, C., Ersser, S., Lloyd, A. and Barnetson, L. (1999) *The Use of Aromatherapy in Intrapartum Midwifery Practice: An evaluative study*, Report no. 7. Oxford: Oxford Centre of Health Care Research and Development, Oxford Brookes University.

Burns, E., Zobbi, V., Panzeri, D., Oskrochi, R. and Regalia, A. (2007) Aromatherapy in childbirth: a pilot randomised controlled trial, *BJOG: An International Journal of Obstetrics and Gynaecology*, 114 (7): 838–44.

Burvill, S. (2002) Midwifery diagnosis of labour onset, *British Journal of Midwifery*, 10 (10): 600–5.

Cesario, S. (2004) Re-evaluation of Friedman's labour curve: a pilot study, *Journal of Obstetrics, Gynaecology and Neonatal Nursing*, 33 (6): 713–22.

Chang, M., Wang, S. and Chen, C. (2002) Effect of massage on pain and anxiety during labour, *Journal of Advanced Nursing*, 38 (1): 68–73.

Chapman, V. (ed.) (2003) *The Midwife's Labour and Birth Handbook*. Oxford: Blackwell Publishing.

Cheyne, H., Dowding, D. and Hundley, V. (2006) Making the diagnosis of labour: midwives' diagnostic judgement and management decisions, *Journal of Advanced Nursing*, 53 (6): 625–35.

Clement, S. (1994) Unwanted vaginal examinations, *British Journal of Midwifery*, 2 (8): 368–70.

Cluett, E. and Burns, E. (2009) Immersion in water in labour, and birth, *Cochrane Database of Systematic Reviews*, 2: CD000111.

Cluett, E., Pickering, R., Getliffe, K. and Saunders, N. (2004) Randomised controlled trial of labouring in water compared with standard of augmentation for management of dystocia in first stage of labour, *British Medical Journal*, 328 (7435): 314–18.

Crowther, C., Enkin, M., Keirse, M. and Brown, I. (2000) Monitoring progress in labor, in M. Enkin, M. Keirse, J. Neilson, C. Crowther, L. Duley, E. Hodnett et al. (eds) *A Guide to Effective Care in Pregnancy and Childbirth* (3rd edn). Oxford: Oxford University Press.

Davies, S. (2011) A longer labour and birth . . . one size does not fit all, in S. Donna (ed.) *Promoting Normal Birth: research, reflections and guidelines*. Chester-le-Street: Fresh Heart Publishing.

Dhany, A., Mitchell, T. and Foy, C. (2012) Aromatherapy and massage intrapartum service impact upon use of analgesia in women in labour: a retrospective case note analysis, *Journal of Alternative and Complementary Medicine*, 18 (10): 932–88.

Dixon, L. and Foureur, M. (2010) The vaginal examination during labour: is it of benefit or harm?, *New Zealand College of Midwives Journal*, 42: 21–6.

Duff, M. (2005) *A study of labour*, unpublished PhD dissertation, University of Technology, Sydney, NSW.

El-Sayed, Y. (2012) Diagnosis and management of arrest disorders: duration to wait, *Seminars in Perinatology*, 36 (5): 374–8.

Eriksson, M., Mattsson, L. and Ladfors, L. (1997) Early or late bath during the first stage of labour: a randomized study of 200 women, *Midwifery*, 13 (3): 146–8.

Field, T. (2010) Pregnancy and labor massage therapy, *Expert Review of Obstetrics and Gynecology*, 5 (2): 177–81.

Field, T., Hernandez-Reif, M., Taylor, S., Quintino, O. and Burman, I. (1997) Labour pain is reduced by massage therapy, *Journal of Psychosomatic Obstetrics and Gynecology*, 18 (4): 286–91.

Foulkes, J. and Dumoulin, J. (1985) The effects of ketonuria in labour, *British Journal of Clinical Practice*, 39 (2): 59–62.

Friedman, E. (1954) The graphic analysis of labour, *American Journal of Obstetrics and Gynecology*, 68 (6): 1568–75.

Gallo, R., Santana, L., Ferreira, C., Marcolin, A. (2013) Massage reduced severity of pain during labour: a randomised controlled trial, *Journal of Physiotherapy*, 59 (2): 109–16.

Garite, T., Weeks, J., Peters-Phair, K., Pattillo, C. and Brewster, W. (2000) A randomized controlled trial of the effect of increased intravenous hydration on the course of labor in nulliparous women, *American Journal of Obstetrics and Gynecology*, 183 (6): 1544–8.

Garland, D. and Jones, K. (2000) Waterbirths: supporting practice with clinical audit, *MIDIRS Midwifery Digest*, 10 (3): 333–6.

Gaskin, I. (2003) Going backwards: the concept of 'pasmo', *The Practising Midwife*, 6 (8): 34–6.

Geissbuehler, V., Stein, S. and Eberhard, J. (2004) Waterbirths compared with landbirths: an observational study of nine years, *Journal of Perinatal Medicine*, 32 (4): 308–14.

Gholitabar, M. (2009) *Why women do not adopt upright positions during labour and birth: an exploratory study*, doctoral thesis, University of West London.

Ginesi, L. and Niescierowicz, R. (1998a) Neuroendocrinology and birth 1: stress, *British Journal of Midwifery*, 6 (10): 659–63.

Ginesi, L. and Niescierowicz, R. (1998b) Neuroendocrinology and birth 2: the role of oxytocin, *British Journal of Midwifery*, 6 (12): 791–6.

Glazener, C., Abdalla, M., Stroud, P., Naji, S., Templeton, A. and Russell, I. (1995) Postnatal maternal morbidity: extent, causes, prevention and treatment, *British Journal of Obstetrics and Gynaecology*, 102 (4): 282–7.

Green, J., Baston, H., Easton, S. and McCormick, F. (2003) *Greater Expectations. Inter-relationships between women's expectations and experiences of decision making, continuity, choice and control in labour, and psychological outcomes*, Summary report. Mother and Infant Research Unit, University of Leeds.

Green, J., Coupland, V. and Kitzinger, J. (1998) *Great Expectations: A prospective study of women's expectations and experiences of childbirth*. Hale: Books for Midwives Press.

Greenberg, M., Cheng, Y., Sullivan, M., Norton, M., Hopkins, L. and Caughey, A. (2007) Does length of labor vary by maternal age?, *American Journal of Obstetrics and Gynecology*, 197 (4): 428.e1–7.

Hall, M. (2001) Caesarean section, in G. Lewis (ed.) *Why Mothers Die 1997–1999*. The Fifth Report of the Confidential Enquiries into Maternal Deaths in the United Kingdom. London: RCOG.

Hobbs, L. (1998) Assessing cervical dilatation without VEs, *The Practising Midwife*, 1 (11): 34–5.

Hodnett, E.D., Gates, S., Hofmeyr, G.J. and Sakala, C. (2013) Continuous support for women during childbirth, *Cochrane Database of Systematic Reviews*, 7: CD003766.

Inch, S. (1985) Management of the third stage of labour: another cascade of intervention?, *Midwifery*, 1 (2): 114–22.

Jay, A. and Hamilton, C. (2008) Intrapartum care, in I. Peate and C. Hamilton (eds) *Becoming a Midwife in the 21st Century*. Chichester: Wiley-Blackwell.

Joy, S. and Peng, T. (2011) Abnormal labour, *Medscape* [http://emedicine.medscape.com/article/273053-overview].

Kabiru, W., Jamieson, D., Graves, W. and Lindsay, M. (2001) Trends in operative vaginal delivery rates and associated maternal complication rates in an inner city hospital, *American Journal of Obstetrics and Gynecology*, 184 (6): 1112–14.

Kennell, J., Klaus, M., McGrath, S., Robertson, S. and Hinkley, C. (1991) Continuous emotional support during labor in a US hospital: a randomized controlled trial, *Journal of the American Medical Association*, 265 (17): 2197–2201.

Khoda Karami, N., Safarzadeh, A. and Fathizadeh, N. (2007) Effect of massage therapy on severity of pain and outcome of labor in primipara, *Iranian Journal of Nursing and Midwifery Research*, 12 (1): 6–9.

Kjærgaard, H., Olsen, J., Ottesen, B. and Dykes, A. (2009) Incidence and outcomes of dystocia in the active phase of labor in term nulliparous women with spontaneous labor onset, *Acta Obstetricia et Gynecologica Scandinavica*, 88 (4): 402–7.

Kumud, Rana, A. and Chopra, S. (2013) Effect of upright positions on the duration of first stage of labour among nulliparous mothers, *Nursing and Midwifery Research Journal*, 9 (1): 10–20.

Lavendar, T., Hart, A. and Smyth, R. (2013) Effect of partogram use on outcomes for women in spontaneous labour at term, *Cochrane Database of Systematic Reviews*, 4: CD005461.

Lawrence, A., Lewis, L., Hofmeyr, G., Dowswell, T. and Styles, C. (2009) Maternal positions and mobility during first stage of labour, *Cochrane Database of Systematic Reviews*, 2: CD003934.

Lee, M., Chang, S. and Kang, D. (2004) Effects of SP6 acupressure on labor pain and length of delivery time in women during labor, *Journal of Alternative and Complementary Medicine*, 10 (6): 959–65.

Liu, E. and Sia, A. (2004) Rates of caesarean section and instrumental vaginal delivery in nulliparous women after low concentration epidural infusions or opioid analgesia: systematic review, *British Medical Journal*, 328 (7453): 1410–16.

Lowe, N. and Corwin, E. (2011) Proposed biological linkages between obesity, stress, and inefficient uterine contractility during labor in humans, *Medical Hypotheses*, 76 (5): 755–60.

Martin, C. (2009) Effects of Valsalva manoeuvre on maternal and fetal wellbeing, *British Journal of Midwifery*, 17 (5): 279–85.

Mendelson, C. (1946) The aspiration of stomach contents into the lungs during obstetric anaesthesia, *American Journal of Obstetrics and Gynecology*, 52: 191–205.

Midwives Information and Resources Service (MIDIRS) (2008) *Positions in Labour and Delivery*, Informed Choice for Professionals Leaflet. Bristol: MIDIRS.

Moneta, J., Okninska, A., Wielgos, M., Przybos, A., Szymusik, I. and Marianowski, L. (2001) Patients' preferences concerning the course of labor, *Ginekologia Polska*, 72 (12): 1010–18.

National Institute for Health and Clinical Excellence (NICE) (2008) *Induction of Labour*, Clinical Guideline CG70. London: NICE.

National Institute for Health and Clinical Excellence (NICE) (2014) *Intrapartum Care: Care of healthy women and their babies during childbirth*. Clinical Guideline CG190. London: NICE.

Neal, J.L., Lowe, N.K., Ahijevych, K.L., Patrick, T.E., Cabbage, L.A. and Corwin. E.J. (2010) 'Active labor' duration and dilation rates among low-risk, nulliparous women with spontaneous labor onset: a systematic review, *Journal of Midwifery and Women's Health*, 55 (4): 308–15.

Nursing and Midwifery Council (NMC) (2012) *Midwives Rules and Standards*. London: NMC.

Nursing and Midwifery Council (NMC) (2015) *The Code: Professional standards of practice and behaviour for nurses and midwives*. London: NMC.

O'Driscoll, K., Jackson, R. and Gallagher, J. (1969) Prevention of prolonged labour, *British Medical Journal*, 2 (5655): 477–80.

O'Mahony, F., Hofmeyr, G. and Menon, V. (2010) Choice of instruments for assisted vaginal delivery, *Cochrane Database of Systematic Reviews*, 11: CD005455.

O'Sullivan, G., Liu, B., Hart, D., Seed, P. and Shennan, A. (2009) Effect of food intake during labor on obstetric outcome: randomized controlled trial COMMENT, *Obstetrical and Gynecological Survey*, 64 (9): 567–8.

Otigbah, C.M., Dhanjal, M.K. and Harmsworth, G. (2000) A retrospective comparison of water births and conventional vaginal deliveries, *European Journal of Obstetrics & Gynecology and Reproductive Biology*, 91 (1): 15–20.

Patel, R. and Murphy, D. (2004) Forceps delivery in modern obstetric practice, *British Medical Journal*, 328 (7451): 1302–5.

Perkins, B. (2004) *The Medical Delivery Business: Health reform, childbirth and the economic order*. London: Rutgers University Press.

Philpott, R. and Castle, W. (1972) Cervicographs in the management of labour of primigravidae: the alert line for detecting abnormal labour, *Journal of Obstetrics and Gynaecology of the British Commonwealth*, 79: 592–8.

Reed, R. (2011) The assessment of progress, *AIMS Journal*, 23 (2): 11–13.

Royal College of Midwives (RCM) (2012a) *Evidenced Based Guidelines for Midwifery-led Care in Labour: Assessing progress in labour*. London: RCM [https://www.rcm.org.uk/sites/default/files/Assessing%20Progress%20in%20Labour.pdf].

Royal College of Midwives (RCM) (2012b) *Evidenced Based Guidelines for Midwifery-led Care in Labour: Nutrition in labour*. London: RCM [https://www.rcm.org.uk/sites/default/files/Nutrition%20in%20Labour.pdf].

Shepherd, A., Cheyne, H., Kennedy, S., McIntosh, C., Styles, M. and Niven, C. (2010) The purple line as a measure of labour progress: a longitudinal study, *BMC Pregnancy and Childbirth*, 10: 54.

Shields, S., Ratcliffe, S., Fontaine, P. and Leeman, L. (2007) Dystocia in nulliparous women, *American Family Physician*, 75 (11): 1671–8.

Simkin, P. and Ancheta, R. (2011) *The Labor Progress Handbook: Early interventions to prevent and treat dystocia* (3rd edn). Chichester: Wiley-Blackwell.

Simkin, P. and O'Hara, M. (2002) Nonpharmacologic relief of pain during labor: systematic reviews of five methods, *American Journal of Obstetrics and Gynecology*, 186 (5 suppl.): S131–59.

Singata, M., Tranmer, J. and Gyte, G. (2010) Restricting oral fluid and food intake during labour, *Cochrane Database of Systematic Reviews*, 1: CD003930.

Skilnand, E., Fossen, D. and Heiberg, E. (2002) Acupuncture in the management of pain in labour, *Acta Obstetricia et Gynecologica Scandinavica*, 81 (10): 943–8.

Smith, C., Levett, K., Collins, C. and Jones, L. (2012) Massage reflexology and other manual methods for pain management in labour, *Cochrane Database of Systematic Reviews*, 2: CD009290.

Smyth, R.M.D., Alldred, S.K. and Markham, C. (2013) Amniotomy for shortening spontaneous labour, *Cochrane Database of Systematic Reviews*, 1: CD006167.

Spiby, H., Green, J., Renfrew, M., Crawshaw, S., Stewart, P., Lishman, J. et al. (2008) *Improving Care at the Primary/Secondary Interface: A trial of community based support in early labour. The ELSA trial*. Report for the National Co-ordinating Centre for the NHS Service Delivery and Organisation R&D (NCCSDO). London: NCCSDO.

Stuart, C. (2000) Invasive actions in labour: where have all the old tricks gone?, *The Practising Midwife*, 3 (8): 30–3.

Thoni, A., Mussner, K. and Ploner, F. (2010) Water birthing: retrospective review of 2625 water births: contamination of birth pool water and risk of microbial cross infection, *Minerva Ginecologica*, 62 (3): 203–11.

Walsh, D. (2010) Labour rhythms, in D. Walsh and S. Downe (eds) *Essential Midwifery Practice: Intrapartum care*. Chichester: Wiley-Blackwell.

Walsh, D. (2011) Care in the first stage of labour, in S. Macdonald and J. Magill-Cuerdon (eds) *Mayes' Midwifery* (14th edn.). London: Ballière Tindall.

Wickham, S. and Sutton, J. (2005) The Rhombus of Michaelis, in S. Wickham (ed.) *Midwifery Best Practice*, Vol. 3. Edinburgh: Elsevier Butterworth-Heinemann.

Zahra, A. and Leila, M. (2013) Lavender aromatherapy massages in reducing labor pain and duration of labor: a randomized controlled trial, *African Journal of Pharmacy and Pharmacology*, 7 (8): 426–30.

Zanetti-Dallenback, R., Tschudin, S., Zhong, X., Holzgreve, W., Lapaire, O. and Hosli, I. (2007) Maternal and neonatal infections and obstetrical outcome in water birth, *European Journal of Obstetrics & Gynecology and Reproductive Biology*, 134 (2): 37–43.

Zhang, J., Troendle, J., Mikolajczyk, R. Sundaram, R., Beaver, J. and Fraser, W. (2010) The natural history of the normal first stage of labor, *American Journal of Obstetrics and Gynecology*, 115 (4): 705–10.

Zhang, J., Troendle, J. and Yanccy, M. (2002) Reassessing the labor curve in nulliparous women, *American Journal of Obstetrics and Gynecology*, 187 (4): 824–8.

Zwelling, E., Johnson, K. and Allen, J. (2006) How to implement complementary therapies for labouring women, *American Journal of Maternal/Child Nursing*, 31 (6): 364–70.

12

Maternal diabetes mellitus and gestational diabetes

Jenny Bailey

Introduction

A woman with maternal diabetes mellitus or gestational diabetes is considered 'high risk' and therefore her pregnancy, labour and birth will be medically managed. In 1996, the World Health Organization (WHO) called for the elimination of unnecessary intervention in childbirth. Although diabetes certainly does warrant medical attention and management, midwives should still support normal physiological processes wherever possible, which includes 'any situation in which the mother feels threatened or unsupported' (ACNM et al., 2012: 66). If childbirth can be normalized or humanized in diabetic women, it will enhance the outcome of both mother and baby. This will require a commitment to shared decision-making on the part of clinicians in an environment where there is time to make decisions free from coercion (ACNM et al., 2012). Having children is a major life decision. Many women who are diabetic do have straightforward pregnancies and give birth to healthy babies, although a lot of dedication and hard work is required on their part. This chapter will discuss these issues and will explore the literature related to gestational diabetes, which remains a controversial topic.

Types of diabetes – and why it is important to know the differences

Diabetes mellitus is a group of metabolic diseases. In 2010 in England, the number of people aged 16 and over with diabetes (diagnosed and undiagnosed) was approximately 3.1 million, accounting for 7.4% of this population (Yorkshire and Humber Public Health Observatory, 2010, cited by NICE, 2012).

There are several types of diabetes, including type I diabetes mellitus, type II diabetes mellitus, maturity-onset diabetes of the young (MODY) and gestational diabetes mellitus (GDM). The general term diabetes tends to be linked to all of the above and should not be confused with a separate condition, diabetes insipidus, which affects the regulation of antidiuretic hormone.

Type I diabetes

Type I diabetes, also known as insulin-dependent diabetes mellitus (IDDM) or juvenile-onset diabetes, is an autoimmune condition where beta cells in the pancreas are destroyed, probably triggered by an assault on the immune system, such as by an infection. It usually presents in young people. The condition results in severely reduced or no insulin production from the pancreas, thus requiring a lifetime of insulin administration. Blood glucose levels are elevated above the norm and the classic clinical signs and symptoms of excessive drinking manifest themselves, due to thirst, frequent micturition and hunger as the body enters starvation mode. Usually, there is no first-degree family history; however, there is a 2–9% chance any offspring will develop the condition, rising to 30% if both parents are affected. Treatment in pregnancy requires continued administration of insulin but usually at a higher level to compensate for the additional 'diabetogenic' effect of pregnancy itself. Occasionally, type I diabetes can develop in adults and is known as latent autoimmune diabetes of adults (LADA); it is often initially misdiagnosed as type II diabetes (see below).

WHO (2013) recommends diabetes mellitus in pregnancy should be diagnosed if one or more of the three criteria listed in Box 12.1 are met.

Box 12.1: WHO (2006) criteria for diabetes mellitus

1   Fasting plasma glucose ≥ 7.0 mmol/L (126 mg/dL)
2   Two-hour plasma glucose ≥ 11.1 mmol/L (200 mg/dL) following a 75 g oral glucose load
3   Random plasma glucose ≥ 11.1 mmol/L (200 mg/dL) in the presence of diabetes symptoms

Type II diabetes

Type II diabetes, also known as non-insulin-dependent diabetes mellitus (NIDDM) or maturity- or adult-onset diabetes, occurs as a result of a gradual decline in beta cell function, leading to insulin deficiency and an increase in resistance to insulin in the target cells of the liver and muscle. The majority of people affected by diabetes mellitus fall into this category. Although genetics plays a role in type II diabetes, it appears to be heavily influenced by environmental factors (Vaxillaire and Froguel, 2006). It is six times more prevalent in South Asian populations and three times more common in African/African-Caribbean peoples.

As can be seen from its alternative names, until recent times it was associated with a mature onset; however, it is now being diagnosed in a much younger population and being linked with a more sedentary lifestyle and raised body mass index (BMI). This can cause confusion over differential diagnosis with other diabetic conditions such as LADA and maturity-onset diabetes of the young (see below).

In pregnancy, type II diabetes is currently treated by diet and exercise, progressing to oral anti-diabetic agents such as metformin if glucose levels are elevated above the norm; some women ultimately are prescribed insulin. The number of people with type II diabetes is set to rise according to NICE (2012). WHO (2011) has now stated that type II diabetes can be diagnosed with a glycated haemoglobin result (HbA1c) as an alternative to the standard glucose measures used. HbA1c levels measure how much glucose has attached to haemoglobin in the previous 120 days (the life span of an erythrocyte). HbA1c levels used to be reported as percentages based on the Diabetes Control and Complications Trial (DCCT). However, in order to standardize values across Europe, they are now reported in units of mmol/mol, in line with the International Federation of Clinical Chemistry (IFCC). A HbA1c value greater than 48 mmol/mol (previously 6.5%) is indicative of type II diabetes.

Maturity-onset diabetes of the young

Maturity-onset diabetes of the young (MODY) is type II diabetes presenting in the under-25s and is an autosomal dominant condition; thus diabetes is present usually in two generations of the same family (Fajans et al., 2001; Spyer, 2008). It is caused by a mutation in one of several known genes, and there are two main forms of MODY: HNF1a/4a and GCK. Although the HNF1a/4a mutation does respond to sulphonamides, insulin will eventually be required. The GCK mutation usually does not progress and no treatment is required. An accurate booking history is essential to ascertain if there is such a history of diabetes in either the woman or the father of the baby.

Practice point

Do you ask about the father's diabetic history and record this in the booking documentation?

In all of the above forms of diabetes, blood glucose levels are higher than the norm. Some types will affect the growth of the fetus whereas others won't. The type of diabetes will also affect the care and treatment regimes of both mother and baby.

Some individuals also display a degree of glucose intolerance, their blood glucose levels being higher than normal but not enough to categorize them as having any specific type of diabetes mellitus.

Gestational diabetes mellitus

Gestational diabetes mellitus (GDM) in pregnancy is a contentious subject. Historically, there has been controversy and ambiguity over the screening and diagnosis of GDM (RCOG, 2011; WHO, 2013). As can be seen from the different types of diabetes mellitus, differential diagnosis is complex when diabetes is diagnosed in pregnancy. This is especially the case if the woman has previously been well, asymptomatic and without the need to visit her general practitioner (GP). Any form of diabetes will be compounded by the additional diabetogenic effect pregnancy causes, altering the true picture of a woman's metabolic state prior to pregnancy. Definitions of gestational diabetes vary and include: a type of diabetes that arises during the second or third trimester of pregnancy (Diabetes UK, 2014); diabetes present in pregnancy that 'usually' resolves following pregnancy; or a 'carbohydrate intolerance of varying degrees of severity with onset or first recognition during pregnancy' (WHO, 1999: 19; Russell et al., 2008). With regard to these three definitions, unless blood glucose returns to normal values by approximately 6 weeks postnatally, it cannot truly be assumed that the woman has been in a diabetic state purely for the duration of the pregnancy.

In 2013, WHO recommended that when hyperglycaemia is first detected at any time in pregnancy, it should be classified as either diabetes mellitus in pregnancy or gestational diabetes mellitus.

Risk factors for gestational diabetes

The NICE guidelines for diabetes in pregnancy (2015) detail a programme targeting biochemical screening to women with risk factors. Box 12.2 lists the risk factors for gestational diabetes and if women 'fit' into any of these categories, they ought to be referred for an oral glucose tolerance test at 28 weeks, or at 16 weeks if GDM has been diagnosed in a previous pregnancy, with a further test at 28 weeks.

Box 12.2: Risk factors for gestational diabetes

- BMI above 30 kg/m²
- Previous macrosomic baby weighing 4.5 kg or more
- Previous gestational diabetes
- Family history of diabetes (first-degree relative with diabetes)
- Family origin with a high prevalence of diabetes:
  - South Asian (specifically women whose country of family origin is India, Pakistan or Bangladesh)
  - Black Caribbean
  - Middle Eastern (specifically women whose country of family origin is Saudi Arabia, United Arab Emirates, Iraq, Jordan, Syria, Oman, Qatar, Kuwait, Lebanon or Egypt)

Source: NICE (2015).

NICE (2015) consider family origin to be a factor for increased risk of gestational diabetes. O'Sullivan et al. (1966, cited by Goer, 1997) undertook a study of diabetic women in pregnancy that consisted of one population of black women and one of white women. Goer commented as early as 1997 that Asian, Hispanic and Native American women have on average higher blood sugars than white or black women and he asserted that if obstetricians were still using O'Sullivan's curve as the normative curve for all pregnant women, then 'some women are being identified as diseased simply because of race'. However, subsequent research has found type II diabetes is more prevalent in these communities, developing at a younger age and progressing much more quickly than in the white population (Department of Health, 2006; Diabetes UK, 2008). It could be argued that an oral glucose tolerance test may identify those women in such communities who have existing type II diabetes rather than GDM.

NICE (2015) also consider a family history of diabetes to be a risk factor for women; as discussed previously, those individuals who have MODY may present with a family history of diabetes. If a woman is categorized as GDM rather than as having MODY and subsequently receives insulin, this could have a detrimental effect on the fetus. A BMI above 30 is also considered a risk factor by NICE, however the transition from obesity to GDM only occurs in a minority of women (Heslehurst et al., 2007).

Glucose tolerance and neonatal outcomes

Women who undergo an oral glucose tolerance test in the UK are diagnosed with gestational diabetes if fasting plasma glucose is $\geq$ 5.6 mmol/L or if the plasma venous glucose concentration is $\geq$ 7.8 mmol/L two hours after the test (NICE, 2015).

The multinational Hyperglycaemia and Pregnancy Outcome (HAPO) Study (Metzger et al., 2008) assessed the relationship of maternal glucose tolerance to neonatal outcomes in 23,000 women. It demonstrated a linear relationship between increased maternal fasting plasma glucose (oral glucose tolerance test at 1 and 2 hours) and birth weight above the 90th centile (Metzger et al., 2008; RCOG, 2011). RCOG (2011) reports additional studies that also confirm this and state that fetal growth can be modified by glucose-lowering therapies, diet and lifestyle interventions. RCOG (2011) cites a randomized control trial undertaken in Australia – The Australian Carbohydrate Intolerance Study in Pregnant Women (ACHOIS) (Crowther et al., 2005) – which established that treatment of gestational diabetes with insulin improved pregnancy outcome. The trial is reported to have used the same definition of gestational diabetes as the 2008a NICE guideline (RCOG, 2011). They also stated that shoulder dystocia was reduced from 4% to 1%. A further study cited by RCOG and undertaken by the Maternal Fetal Medicines Unit (MFMU) Network Trial used a similar design to ACHOIS but used a definition of gestational diabetes that included lower levels of fasting plasma glucose (< 5.3 mmol/L) and postprandial thresholds at 2 and 3 hours (Landon et al., 2009). The only significant outcome was a reduction in birth weight of 106 g in infants weighing over 4 kg. Other outcomes were not statistically significant.

Screening and treatment for diabetes

As a result of a number of study trials, the International Association of Diabetes and Pregnancy Study Group (IADSPG, 2010) reconsidered the diagnosis of and screening for diabetes in a consensus report. This group suggest that women who require pharmacological intervention should initially be prescribed oral hypoglycaemic agents (metformin or glibenclamide) and then progress to insulin to ensure adequate glycaemic control. They state that this regime is as successful as but not better than the use of insulin alone with regard to immediate pregnancy outcomes. There is a very real concern, therefore, that if blood glucose levels cannot be controlled by diet and exercise, then some obstetricians may well inappropriately manage the condition with insulin, omitting the oral hypoglycaemic agent stage altogether. While this approach may be to the benefit of neonates, the potential impact and implications for childbearing women and maternity services are immense. There is a move for NICE and therefore England and Wales to adopt the international consensus findings in the near future. Whereas at present NICE (2015) have identified risk factors to be identified prior to an oral glucose tolerance test at 28 weeks, if adopted all women would undergo such screening at 24–28 weeks gestation.

The implications of changes to screening criteria for gestational diabetes

If the ACHOIS criteria are adopted, then it is predicted that rates of gestational diabetes per pregnancy in the UK will rise from 3.5% to 16% (RCOG, 2011). As a consequence, many more women will be labelled as 'gestational diabetics'. The RCOG state that: 'the interventions proposed for women with gestational diabetes are relatively non-invasive in most women and have an effect on both new born weight and maternal weight gain' (2011: 4).

With the population of women with GDM increasing to 16% and approximately 8–20% of these women requiring insulin (RCOG, 2011), it could be argued that significantly more pregnant women will be injecting insulin. This is an invasive procedure and carries with it its own risk of morbidity and potential fatality due to error of administration. With regard to fetal macrosomia in GDM, treatment with insulin caused a reduction of only 106 g; this is negligible with regard to birth trauma in a baby weighing more than 4 kg. Goer questioned whether it is right to justify 'manipulating the growth mechanism of babies, roughly 75–80% of who will fall below the 90th percentile for weight if left alone' (1997: 175). Other authors have stated that prediction of fetal macrosomia is poor when based on factors such as GDM, BMI, parity and age (Jolly et al., 2003).

For women who present with GDM of unclear aetiology and if insulin was used to treat, it could severely compromise those fetuses that acquire the GCK mutation from their mothers if they have MODY (Spyer, 2008). Other fetuses may become small for gestational age (SGA) due to insulin administration. One can therefore surmise that this will also require further interventions, such as: increased surveillance, potential iatrogenic preterm labour and associated risks with the small for gestational age baby.

If more women undergo insulin therapy and as a consequence have their labour medically managed, this is also likely to have an impact on induction, augmentation of labour and caesarean section rates. The financial implications of an increase in the number of midwives needed to provide the necessary one-to-one care, medicines and equipment and of caesarean section compared with normal birth have yet to be considered if this change to the current screening programme proceeds.

For many women, being pregnant is the first time they have prolonged contact with health services, when they may be required to have intensive screening and monitoring. If the UK does follow ACHOIS guidelines and a 75 g oral glucose tolerance test is administered to all women at 24–28 weeks gestation, and if their blood glucose levels are elevated, initially it would be difficult to ascertain a differential diagnosis of previously undiagnosed type I or type II diabetes, LADA or MODY. A confirmatory diagnosis could not be undertaken until the postnatal test was performed. The increased workload that would be created for the medical staff could potentially be off-loaded to midwives running diabetic clinics if there is a rise of 3.5–16% in the number of women diagnosed.

Given that the numbers of women with types I and II diabetes are rising both nationally and internationally, that there is an increase in obesity and women are having babies later in life in the UK, then a 16% pregnant population with GDM may be a conservative estimate. This also means that even less women will experience continuity of care with their community midwives, as these women will all be referred to the hospital-based consultant-led team.

WHO (2013) recommends that the diagnosis of gestational diabetes should be based on any of the criteria listed in Box 12.3.

Box 12.3: WHO (2013) criteria for gestational diabetes

1   Fasting plasma glucose of 5.1–6.9 mmol/L (92–125 mg/dL)
2   One-hour plasma glucose ≥ 10.0 mmol/L (180 mg/dL)* following a 75 g oral glucose load
3   Two-hour plasmas glucose of 8.5–11.0 mmol/L (153–199 mg/dL) following a 75 g oral glucose load

_____

*There are no established criteria for the diagnosis of diabetes mellitus based on the one-hour post-load value (see Box 12.1).

WHO (2013) recognize that the quality of evidence for these criteria is very low and therefore it is considered a weak recommendation.

Medical management of diabetes and considerations for more woman-centred care

In the 2001 National Service Framework (NSF) for Diabetes, the Department of Health stated:

> The NHS will develop, implement and monitor policies that seek to empower and support women with pre-existing diabetes and those who develop diabetes during pregnancy to optimise outcomes of their pregnancy.
>
> (Department of Health, 2001: 5)

In 2008, Diabetes UK reported that women were not receiving the care they needed and more progress was required to achieve the NSF standards set in 2001. No national data are routinely collected in relation to the provision of pre-pregnancy and pregnancy services for women with diabetes. NICE (2015) have produced guidelines for the management of diabetes and its complications from preconception to the postnatal period (2015).

Preconception care

NICE (2015) state the importance of avoiding unplanned pregnancy in women with diabetes and suggest that women be offered appropriate advice prior to discontinuing contraception. Women with diabetes should be guided in optimal glycaemic control and provided with relevant advice, such as taking folic acid 5 mg daily prior to pregnancy and for up to 12 weeks antenatally. This is because high levels of glucose can interfere with embryological and fetal neuchal cord development. Ideally, midwives should be involved in preconception care. In reality, however, most women see the diabetic specialist midwife once they are pregnant and have been referred to the diabetic clinic for pregnant mothers.

Practice points

The following points were designed with community midwives in mind.

- Do your local health centres hold diabetic clinics for childbearing women?
- Do you know the local practice and diabetic nurses who usually run these clinics?
- Have you considered joint preconception care clinics with the practice/ diabetic nurses at your GP surgeries?

Preconception advice is extremely important for women with diabetes and more user-friendly ways of delivering this information can be adopted. For example, Diabetes UK's website has two excellent short videos about living with type I diabetes as an adolescent – 'Rebel Rebel' and 'Top preconception tips from

Becca'. The links to these can be found in the 'Useful websites' section at the end of the chapter.

Women need to be engaged with their pregnancy and diabetes. Queen's University Belfast also has a series of mini videos for women to access, some that come with mini quizzes the women can interact with (see the 'Useful websites' section). Perhaps more information using social media could be used to engage women in their care. The 'Birth I want' initiative on Facebook is an example of a discursive space where knowledge and power might emerge from such forums.

The DAFNE (Dose Adjustment for Normal Eating) programme provides those over 17 with type I diabetes with the skills necessary to estimate carbohydrate intake at each meal. The programme has a website and an app can be downloaded that enables women to store their recordings online in a diary. The website also has a number of forums and useful carbohydrate portion lists for quick and easy access (again, see the 'Useful websites' section).

Practice points

- Does your unit have a website or Facebook page that women can access for help and advice?
- Do you use blogs, tweets or texts? If you do, are they also in other languages?

Antenatal care

Regarding antenatal care for women with diabetes, NICE (2015) state that general information about pregnancy and birth should be covered during antenatal appointments, as it is with women who do not have diabetes. Women who are pregnant and have a chronic illness often experience information overload, the majority of which is about their chronic condition rather than specifically about pregnancy. Although many women with a chronic condition become pregnant, little is known about what pregnancy is like for these women. In a small qualitative study by Tyer-Viola and Lopez (2014), a common theme expressed by the women was that of maintaining a balancing act. The analogy of the tension of being on a high wire was used to describe trying to be normal (like any other pregnant woman) while balancing this against simultaneously managing a chronic illness while pregnant. This balancing act caused some women stress. Levels of stress biomarkers such as cortisol and corticotrophin releasing hormone (CRH) can lead to preterm birth (McCoy et al., 2008; Yim et al., 2009), which exacerbates physical morbidity in the woman, the fetus and baby of the woman with diabetes. Therefore, reducing women's stress levels should be a priority. In Tyer-Viola and Lopez's (2014) study, women spent a considerable amount of time thinking about how pregnancy affected their condition and about potential outcomes, and thus some felt they couldn't get too excited about their pregnancy, and found it to be an emotional burden. There was a balance to be made between celebrating being pregnant and handling knowing about potential sequelae both for herself and her baby. The women very much longed to be normal and some were envious of women who did not have a chronic illness and queried why those women complained about the usual clinical manifestations of pregnancy. Seeking information about pregnancy always came with a disclaimer and healthcare professionals often drew them back from the dream of a normal pregnancy towards the reality of potential complications in the forthcoming weeks. One woman stated:

> Like, I'm another normal pregnant lady coming for a doctor's check up, but unfortunately there's more times than not that I walked out of those appointments in tears because of complications that kept coming up and all these fears that arise.
>
> (Tyer-Viola and Lopez, 2014: 33)

Some women dealt with the stress and anxiety through what Tyer-Viola and Lopez (2014) call 'protective governing', whereby they tried to put a positive spin on things, seeing their concerns as related to a normal event – being pregnant. In order to help reduce stress and worry, Tyer-Viola and Lopez suggest that milestones reached to date be acknowledged in consultations, which allows subsequent care to be put into context. They also suggest follow-up phone calls 24 hours after each appointment to review information and help allay fears.

Practice points

- Do you provide positive encouragement regarding milestones reached?
- Does your unit undertake follow-up phone calls to review information?
- Do you have a dedicated phone line for women to discuss any issues regarding their care?

If a woman has pre-existing diabetes or develops diabetes in pregnancy, she ought to be referred to the specialist team either by the midwife or GP. As a result, input from the community midwife is reduced or lost altogether because the majority of the antenatal appointments are undertaken with the specialist team in a secondary care hospital environment. This is a missed opportunity for the woman to be treated like any other pregnant woman. For women with pre-existing diabetes and used to the specialist team input, the increased surveillance may reinforce the fact that she is a diabetic woman who is pregnant rather than a pregnant woman with diabetes. The joy of her pregnancy may well be quashed.

Case 12.1: Rachel

At 28 weeks gestation, I had a glucose tolerance test that was 'slightly over the normal level'. From this point on my care changed. I no longer had midwife appointments and instead went to the fetal care unit for a diabetes clinic every two weeks. These appointments were very different to the other care I'd received, and the focus became primarily about the four times daily glucose readings. I was never weighed, measured or asked about my general wellbeing, and never got to hear baby's heart beat. Luckily, my readings were always well within the normal range and there was no cause for concern. But our conversations were still always focused on risk to the baby during the pregnancy and impending birth. I asked to be discharged back to midwifery care after 4–5 weeks but was told once I was 'on the pathway' that I had to remain there, as that was the protocol.

Everything was prescriptive. The birth had to happen in the labour ward rather than the very good birthing unit that was just next door. I was to be induced at 38 weeks, which I negotiated back to 39 weeks with some difficulty – the doctor I saw during that meeting handed me a copy of the NICE guidelines for managing diabetes in pregnancy, which I found very scary!

Care and attention related to my baby's wellbeing before and after his birth were exceptional. What frustrated me was the lack of flexibility when it came to the care pathway. Staff did not seem able to use their clinical judgement. The diabetes tainted what was otherwise a perfect pregnancy. I felt extremely well throughout, was active and eating healthily.

During labour, I was at home with a doula and then arrived at hospital 8 cm dilated. I was pushing within an hour of arriving. With 'diabetes' written across all of my notes, the staff followed the protocol to the letter and I was hooked up to a monitor right away and put in a reclined position despite my doula's protests. My contractions were overwhelming at this point and I'd had no pain relief, so I very much went along with it. I had blood glucose readings taken – again, even though I'd not had an abnormal result for months, which seemed like total overkill.

The fetal heart rate became a cause for concern. A lot of people arrived very quickly, and my baby was delivered by emergency forceps after a failed attempt at a ventouse. It was overwhelming and although the staff tried to stay calm, it was quite frightening. I am extremely grateful for the quick thinking of the staff there on that day but my baby's entry into the world was harsh, brutal and left us both with scars – physical and emotional. I sustained a third-degree tear, and despite very good follow-up support from the surgeon and a physio, this took its toll physically in the early weeks and months.

Following the birth there was a focus on glucose monitoring for both of us. While in theatre having a third-degree repair, our baby was bottle-fed by my husband on the insistence of the staff, and as breastfeeding was going badly when I returned the emphasis again became on 'getting the baby fed' so his levels didn't drop. Everything was focused on preventing a problem rather than treating a mother and baby who were well and healthy. If I could go back and do it again

I would ask for a re-test, as I truly believe the test results may have been flawed somehow. Again, all the evidence suggested there was no diabetes at all, yet staff were insistent that they couldn't deviate from a very strict protocol.

This medicalized pathway meant that I grieved for the proactive, natural birth I had hoped for. I analysed those final moments of delivery for many months – asking myself if I had not been seen as a 'diabetic' mother, would the staff have done anything differently. Our inability to breastfeed was even more painful and I strongly feel this was down to the staff's insistence on bottle-feeding, and their unwillingness to wait and see for a few hours.

I've since gone on to have another health 6-lb baby boy, and second time around was not diagnosed with gestational diabetes.

With thanks to Rachel

Obstetricians and diabetic specialist midwives may wish to review the use of satellite clinics in the community and at GP surgeries, and in maintaining the community midwife contact as per NICE antenatal guidelines (2008b) in addition to specialist team input.

Finding out you have diabetes in pregnancy must be very alarming, and the wishes and aspirations for pregnancy and childbirth that these women have may well be lost in the ensuing 'cascade of intervention' (Inch, 1985). In the third stage of labour that Inch was referring to, the cascade is likely to involve medical and associated professionals with the possible exclusion of the midwife. For some women, it may mean they cannot have the pregnancy and birth they had hoped for. Diabetes has an impact on people's lives and can affect their careers, driving and insurance policies. Some people who have been diagnosed as having diabetes feel they have been condemned to a life where everything has to be planned (Burden, 2003).

Community midwives should ensure that they arrange additional appointments with diabetic women outside their specialist clinic consultations to discuss the pregnancy and any other issues that arise; this may also help with reducing stress levels and provide the women with some sense of normality – something which they crave.

The majority of multidisciplinary diabetic clinics do not have a midwife present (CEMACH, 2007). When midwives are present, they usually take an administrative role and direct women to the various members of the specialist team to be seen as part of the medical management (dietician, ultrasonographer, diabetic and obstetric consultants). There is the risk that in 'midwifery-led' diabetic clinics, the midwife rarely has the opportunity to see and speak with the woman about usual pregnancy concerns or advocate on her behalf. This is due to the fact that the midwife is involved in the running and administration of the clinic rather than providing midwifery care and information to women.

Women often see medical management of diabetes as a set of instructions they must follow if they are to minimize potential complications such as maternal and fetal morbidity/mortality. This can be very frightening and it also goes against the principles of the Department of Health NHS Plan (2000), whereby women should be actively involved in decision-making.

Records of blood glucose tests and urinalysis are usually kept in a 'log' book, which is completed at each clinic visit; this may be viewed as being more akin to being monitored in a laboratory. Perhaps a more modern approach could be used with some women, including using texts or apps such as the Diabetes UK app. This would be particularly relevant to today's young women. Blog pages could be set up to address issues and answer questions much more quickly than having to wait for the next clinic or having to phone. And the language used in information leaflets could be written in a friendlier and more compassionate way, perhaps inviting women for further screening rather than telling them to attend.

NICE guidelines (2015) also state: all women using insulin or glibenclamide are to maintain their capillary blood glucose above 4 mmol/L. In addition, NICE recommend women maintain the fasting and postprandial capillary plasma glucose levels shown in Box 12.4.

Box 12.4: NICE capillary blood glucose levels for women with diabetes in the antenatal period

1   Fasting capillary plasma glucose of 5.3 mmol/L (95.4 mg/dL)
2   One-hour postprandial capillary plasma glucose of 7.8 mmol/L (140.4 mg/dL)
3   Two-hour postprandial capillary plasma glucose of 6.4 mmol/L (115.2 mg/dL)

Source: NICE (2015).

Common practice is to closely monitor the postprandial recordings, as this is a better predictor of how well diabetes is being controlled.

Blood glucose levels should be kept low in pregnancy so long as it is not to the detriment of maternal wellbeing. The 'Why Mothers Die' report of 2000–2002 (Temple, 2008) recorded three deaths secondary to hypoglycaemia. In the latest CMACE report, 'Saving Mothers' Lives' (CMACE, 2011), a further three women were recorded as dying, the deaths being attributed to probable hypoglycaemia. Hypoglycaemia begets hypoglycaemia: if women are exposed to recurrent hypoglycaemic attacks, physiologically a subsequent worsening state is required before the clinical symptoms of hypoglycaemia become apparent to them, predisposing them to further hypoglycaemic attacks, and this worsens mid-pregnancy (Temple, 2008).

A nationwide study of IDDM in the first trimester (Evers et al., 2002) together with other studies looking at hypoglycaemia in pregnancy (Nielsen et al., 2008; Temple, 2008) show that 50% of women with IDDM have at least one severe hypoglycaemic attack and 10% of women have more than five episodes of severe hypoglycaemia. In both cases, 80% of the attacks occur before 20 weeks gestation.

Worryingly, 52% occur during sleep and 37% during the night. The use of pumps may help reduce these rates in the future (see below). Women should be sensitively informed of this fact and encouraged to keep glucose drinks, sweets and biscuits by the bedside for such an emergency. NICE (2015) also recommend that bedtime target plasma glucose levels ought to be agreed with women who are taking insulin. This level should take into account timing of the last meal and its related insulin dose, and the level should also be consistent with the recommended fasting level on waking (5–7 mmol/L, or 90–126 mg/dL).

The most committed of women struggle to achieve the glucose levels set by NICE (2015). It is better that some women keep their glucose levels slightly higher than optimum rather than suffer recurrent hypoglycaemic attacks with the associated adverse effects on mortality and morbidity of both mother and fetus. Women are not necessarily informed of this compromise, with the emphasis placed firmly on achieving the set targets, leading to a sense of failure and/or a recurrence of hypoglycaemic attacks.

With a growing diabetic population, insulin pumps may become the norm meaning women no longer have to inject several bolus doses of insulin each day. To date there has been no randomized controlled trial to support the use of pumps in pregnancy (Temple, 2008), although anecdotally more women appear to be using them, particularly women with uncontrolled diabetes despite multiple single-dose injections. It offers them stability, independence and autonomy. Currently, they are very expensive although women can apply for funding to help meet the cost. Although the development of insulin pumps is in its infancy, improvements are being made. A link to the use of insulin pumps on the Diabetes UK website is provided at the end of the chapter.

Most women with diabetes are usually induced at 38 weeks of pregnancy, though women with well-controlled gestational diabetes mellitus (controlled by diet and exercise) may wish to await spontaneous onset of labour.

Intrapartum care

Currently, most women with diabetes who require an insulin sliding scale regime during labour are kept relatively inert in their birthing beds due to the array of equipment, electric pumps and infusions. It is well documented that reduced mobility slows the birth process (Lawrence et al., 2009). A little lateral thinking by midwives will keep these women mobile during labour or at least help them to try and adopt natural birth positions. Insulin pumps, such as those noted in the previous section, may be of benefit here, as they work independently via batteries and are very small. They are secured by tape so that they do not become dislodged despite the wearer being active. They negate the requirement for the associated dextrose intravenous infusion (though it may be advisable to still have a cannula *in situ*). By using such pumps (rather than infusion pumps, which need to be plugged into the electricity supply), midwives can support women to achieve their chosen birth positions. This is still possible with women who have the electric insulin pump; it will just require the midwife to review the ergonomics of the birthing room. If continuous fetal monitoring is required, the woman can still adopt positions on the floor, on a chair or Combi-Trac, or use a birthing ball. Women do not have to be immobile on a bed. The site of the insertion point of the pump can be changed (usually it is in the abdomen) and if used with telemetry for fetal monitoring, women could have pool labours and/or births (using pool birth guidelines). Regarding pool births, most maternity units' policy guidelines exclude women with any form of diabetes, including gestational diabetes. This seems rather short-sighted, particularly if the woman has gestational diabetes where diabetic control is by diet, exercise and oral hypoglycaemic agents.

There are no contra-indications for the use of aromatherapy in women who have diabetes; therefore, existing guidelines can be applied as normal.

Case 12.2: Angela

Angela, aged 34, was 38 weeks pregnant and a type I diabetic; her diabetes was well controlled throughout pregnancy by insulin injections. She came into the labour suite in spontaneous labour as her contractions had commenced 4 hours previously. She had said that she would like to be as mobile as possible and wanted to have a natural birth, if all remained well. The baby was continuously monitored and she had a sliding scale insulin pump and an intravenous infusion of dextrose. Angela expressed her concerns saying that she was worried that all of the tubes and wires may have prevented her from being mobile and adopting natural birth positions. The midwife supporting Angela assured her that after the infusions had been sited and external fetal monitoring commenced, the room layout would be changed. The midwife pushed the bed alongside the wall near to where the electricity supply was, but lowered it and placed the pillows along the back so that it resembled a couch and was used as such. This allowed for cables and wires to reach. A floor mat and birthing ball were also brought in and Angela was shown how she could use the ball on the floor or bed. The midwife asked Angela if she would like a hand massage to calm and relax her.

Practice point

In your own practice, would you have the confidence to support a woman in this way?

Postnatal care

It is important that women have slightly higher than normal blood glucose levels in the postnatal period to prevent hypoglycaemic attacks while caring for their new baby. Insulin requirements fall dramatically after birth and women should reduce their requirements as necessary immediately following the birth. The reported increased risk of maternal hypoglycaemia while breastfeeding can be avoided by eating a small snack prior to the feed. For women with gestational diabetes mellitus (GDM) and type II diabetes, insulin should be stopped immediately after the birth (NICE, 2015).

NICE guidelines (2015) state that lifestyle advice for women with GDM should be provided and that they be offered a plasma glucose measurement test (not an oral glucose tolerance test) 6–13 weeks postnatally and annually thereafter. Women should be informed that a different diagnosis to gestational diabetes may be given following this postnatal test, as a true diagnosis of gestational diabetes can only be made once the blood glucose levels return to normal following pregnancy. If levels do not return to non-pregnant values, then the woman will have another type of diabetes that was not diagnosed prior to the pregnancy but was identified during pregnancy.

Neonatal care

Babies of women with diabetes should be kept with their mothers whenever possible. It is important that after so much medical intervention and so many concerns raised regarding neonatal outcome, the mother is allowed time with her baby. This is a positive reaffirmation that she has done her very best for her baby and that the 'fantasy of normality' can be realized in this instance. Skin-to-skin contact between mother and baby will enhance these feelings of normality. The conduction of heat from the mother will also keep baby warm and help maintain glucose levels to some degree, as energy is not expended trying to keep warm. However, it is normal for blood glucose levels in the newborn to drop below 2 mmol/L within the first 6 hours of birth and following this there is a brisk ketogenic response, triggering glucose production in the baby (de Rooy, 2008). Babies can withstand low blood glucose, as the neonatal brain only requires 30% of adult requirements and additional compensatory mechanisms are in place to protect it from such low glucose (de Rooy, 2008). Thus there is no need to routinely undertake blood glucose monitoring in the first few hours after birth. Infant feeding policies should indicate that the baby is fed within 30 minutes and the first blood glucose reading should not be undertaken until 2–3 hours after the first feed.

Practice points

- Do you encourage skin-to-skin contact immediately or within 30 minutes of birth if the baby is well?
- Do you encourage this in women who have had an instrumental or caesarean section birth?
- Do you feel confident enough to wait until after the second feed (approximately 4 hours later) to undertake blood glucose monitoring of the baby?

Babies of women who have poor glycaemic control in pregnancy can have raised glucose levels themselves and some will have hyperinsulinaemia. For these babies, hypoglycaemia is more prolonged and more severe. For babies with transient hypoglycaemia and a family history of MODY, it would be prudent to ask about the father's diabetic history so that a diagnosis can be made for the infant. Babies of women with diabetes should feed as soon as possible after birth (within 30 minutes) and then at frequent intervals (every 2–3 hours) until pre-feed blood glucose levels are maintained at a minimum of 2.0 mmol/L (NICE, 2015). It is imperative to cease blood glucose monitoring of the baby once results are normal.

The type of feed does modulate metabolic adaptation, with breastfed babies having the ability to compensate for lower blood glucose better than formula-fed babies (de Rooy, 2008). It is essential that babies of women with diabetes are put to the breast as soon as possible. Breastfeeding promotes successful neonatal metabolic adaptation due to suckling ketogenesis and should be the nutrition of choice for these babies (de Rooy, 2008). It should start as soon as possible and the breast should be offered at frequent intervals thereafter. Expressed colostrum and breast milk can also be offered; it is good practice for the community midwife or midwives in the diabetic clinic to teach hand expression from 34 weeks gestation. This colostrum can be frozen and saved and used postnatally between regular offerings of the breast. Once milk is being produced, continued expression between feeds can ensure the baby is topped up, should this be required.

Many barriers to breastfeeding have been reported. There is a higher than average caesarean section rate among women who are diabetic (CEMACH, 2007) and this potentially reduces the ability for skin-to-skin contact and early feeding. A 2007 CEMACH report also highlighted that two-thirds of babies were admitted to the neonatal unit for potentially avoidable reasons and of those babies 82% were inappropriately fed with formula milk as their first feed. This potentiates the risk of abnormal metabolic adaptation. A 'circle of defence and line of authority' is the analogy used by Sherridan (2013: 95) to describe breastfeeding peer counsellors' support for women versus the support provided by healthcare professionals. Rather than women having to be protected from lines of authority, midwives should ensure that a circle of support for feeding is prevalent.

Practice point

Do you feel confident encouraging women with diabetes to put the baby to the breast or offer expressed colostrum or breast milk rather than a formula feed?

Case 12.3: Emma

Emma wanted to breastfeed her baby Jake who was born 40 minutes previously by elective caesarean section. After Jake was born and while still in theatre, the midwife put Jake next to Emma for them to enjoy some skin-to-skin contact.

Emma was in the recovery area with Jake and the midwife was helping her to attach Jake to the breast to feed. Emma had brought with her some stored expressed colostrum for Jake to have were he not to feed well initially. Despite Jake being put to the breast, he was not interested in feeding. The midwife decided to give Jake 2 mL of the expressed colostrum by syringe while next to the breast. The midwife suggested to Emma that they should encourage Jake to go back to the breast if he showed an interest to do so within the next 3 hours. Emma was worried that Jake's blood sugar may be low, but the midwife reassured Emma that the 2 mL of expressed colostrum was sufficient for now and that Jake's blood glucose would not need checking for about another 3 hours.

Practice points

- How comfortable are you about helping women achieve skin-to-skin contact while still in theatre?
- What would give you the confidence to delay undertaking blood glucose screening on Jake until almost 4 hours after his birth?

What do women want?

Stenhouse et al. (2013) found that women want an empathic approach to their pregnancy and for the pregnancy itself to be the focus of attention not the diabetes. An example of such medicalization of pregnancy is guidance on the Diabetes UK website entitled 'the management of pregnant women with diabetes' – surely it is the diabetes that requires managing and not the pregnant woman, and all too often the woman does feel 'managed'.

In Stenhouse and colleagues' (2013) study, women wanted positive encounters with healthcare professionals, but most women had experienced negative encounters with the specialist team and they wanted their own expertise of their diabetic condition to be recognized. In addition, the women felt that healthcare professionals did not seem to value their expertise and own insight into their condition.

Conclusion

The NHS Plan (Department of Health, 2000) expounded the value of people becoming active participants and decision-makers in their own care, rather than recipients of health interventions from health professionals. All too often, childbearing women with diabetes do not to feel involved in decisions concerning their care and not offered the choices 'low-risk' pregnant women are given. Complications exist for women with diabetes and their babies that need to be monitored and preventative strategies and treatment regimens put in place. However, any decisions regarding care should be taken in conjunction with the mother and her family and not forced upon her.

Careful consideration should be given to how information is delivered to women with diabetes, making it more user-friendly and accessible via modern technology and social media. Women who are diabetic need affirmation of milestones reached and the opportunity to review information provided. They want to feel like pregnant women with diabetes not diabetic women who are pregnant. They want to enjoy being pregnant rather than constantly worrying about their diabetes.

Midwives need to be flexible in their approach to providing care to minimize any effects of the routine application of medicalized policies. Wherever possible midwives should facilitate a normal pregnancy and birth experience similar to that provided to women who are deemed to be 'low risk'. It should also be remembered that the majority of babies born to women with diabetes are healthy and well.

Useful websites

Diabetes UK: see the videos 'Rebel Rebel' and 'Top preconception tips from Becca' [http://www.diabetes.org.uk/Guide-to-diabetes/Living_with_diabetes/Pregnancy/]; see also the insulin pumps section [http://www.diabetes.org.uk/Guide-to-diabetes/Teens/Me-and-my-diabetes/Getting-my-glucose-right/Pumps/].

Dose Adjustment for Normal Eating (DAFNE) website [http://www.dafne.uk.com/].

Queen's University Belfast: see the 'Women with diabetes' information site [http://www.qub.ac.uk/elearning/public/WomenWithDiabetesThingsYouNeedToKnow/].

References

American College of Nurse-Midwives, Midwives Alliance of North America and National Association of Certified Professional Midwives (2012) *Supporting healthy and normal physiologic childbirth: a consensus statement by ACNM, MANA, and NAPCM* [http://mana.org/pdfs/Physiological-Birth-Consensus-Statement.pdf].
Burden, M. (2003) Diabetes: signs, symptoms and making a diagnosis, *Nursing Times*, 99 (1): 30–2.
Centre for Maternal and Child Enquiries (CMACE) (2011) Saving mothers' lives – Reviewing maternal deaths to make motherhood safer: 2006–2008. The Eighth Report of the confidential enquiries into maternal deaths in the United Kingdom, *BJOG: An International Journal of Obstetrics and Gynaecology*, 118 (suppl. 1): 1–203.
Confidential Enquiry into Maternal and Child Health (CEMACH) (2007) *Diabetes in Pregnancy: Are we providing the best care? Findings of a national enquiry: England, Wales and Northern Ireland*. London: CEMACH.
Crowther, C.A., Hiller, J.E., Moss, J.R., McPhee, A.J., Jeffries, W.S. and Robinson, J.S. (2005) Effect of treatment of gestational diabetes mellitus on pregnancy outcomes, *New England Journal of Medicine*, 352 (24): 2477–86.
Department of Health (2000) *The NHS Plan: A plan for investment, a plan for reform*. London: TSO.
Department of Health (2001) *National Service Framework for Diabetes: Standards*. London: Department of Health.

Department of Health (2006) *Care Planning in Diabetes: Report from the joint Department of Health and Diabetes UK Care Planning Working Group.* London: Department of Health.

de Rooy, L. (2008) Metabolic fuels for the newborn of the mother with diabetes, in *Diabetes in Pregnancy: The scientific basis for clinical practice.* Educational launch of the NICE guideline 'Diabetes in Pregnancy', 7–8 April 2008, RCOG, London.

Diabetes UK (2008) *The National Service Framework (NSF) for Diabetes: Five years on . . . are we half way there?* London: Diabetes UK [http://www.diabetes.org.uk/Documents/Reports/Five_years_on__are_we_half_way_there2008.pdf; accessed 2 June 2014].

Diabetes UK (2014) *Guide to Diabetes.* London: Diabetes UK [http://www.diabetes.org.uk/Guide-to-diabetes/What-is-diabetes/Other-types-of-diabetes/Gestational-diabetes/; accessed 23 September 2014].

Evers, I.M., ter Braak, E.W., de Valk, H.W., van Der Schoot, B., Janssen, N. and Visser, G.H. (2002) Risk indicators predictive for severe hypoglycaemia during the first trimester of type 1 diabetic pregnancy, *Diabetes Care,* 25 (3): 554–9.

Fajans, S.S., Bell, G.I. and Polonsky, K.S. (2001) Molecular mechanisms and clinical pathophysiology of maturity onset diabetes of the young, *New England Journal of Medicine,* 345 (13): 971–80.

Goer, H. (1997) Gestational diabetes: the emperor has no clothes, *MIDIRS Midwifery Digest,* 7 (2): 173–7.

HAPO Study Cooperative Research Group (2009) Hyperglycaemia and adverse pregnancy outcome (HAPO) study: associations with neonatal anthropometrics, *Diabetes,* 58 (2): 453–9.

Heslehurst, N., Lang, R., Rankin, J., Wilkinson, J.R. and Summerbell, C.D. (2007) Obesity in pregnancy: a study of the impact of maternal obesity on NHS maternity services, *BJOG: An International Journal of Obstetrics and Gynaecology,* 114 (3): 334–42.

Inch, S. (1985) Management of the third stage of labour: another cascade of intervention?, *Midwifery,* 1 (2): 114–22.

International Association of Diabetes and Pregnancy Study Groups (IADPSG) Consensus Panel (2010) Recommendations on the diagnosis and classification of hyperglycaemia in pregnancy, *Diabetes Care,* 33 (3): 676–82.

Jolly, M.C., Sebire, N.J., Harris, J.P., Regan, L. and Robinson, S. (2003) Risk factors for macrosomia and its clinical consequences: a study of 350 311 pregnancies, *European Journal of Obstetrics & Gynaecology and Reproductive Biology,* 111 (1): 9–14.

Landon, M.B., Spong, C.Y., Thom, E., Carpenter, M.W., Ramin, S.M., Casey, B. et al. (2009) A multicenter, randomized trial of treatment for mild gestational diabetes, *New England Journal of Medicine,* 361 (14): 1339–48.

Lawrence, A., Lewis, L., Hofmeyr, G.J., Dowswell, T. and Styles, C. (2009) Maternal positions and mobility during first stage labour, *Cochrane Database of Systematic Reviews,* 2: CD003934.

McCoy, S.J., Beal, J.M., Saunders, B., Hill, E.A., Payton, M.E. and Watson, G.H. (2008) Risk factors for postpartum depression: a retrospective investigation, *Journal of Reproductive Medicine,* 53 (3): 166–70.

Metzger, B.E., Lowe, L.P., Dyer, A.R., Trimble, E.R., Chaovarindr, U., Coustan, D.R. et al. (2008) Hyperglycaemia and adverse pregnancy outcome, *New England Journal of Medicine,* 358 (19): 1991–2002.

National Institute for Health and Clinical Excellence (NICE) (2008a) *Diabetes in Pregnancy,* Clinical Guideline CG63. London: NICE [https://www.nice.org.uk/guidance/cg63].

National Institute for Health and Clinical Excellence (NICE) (2008b) *Antenatal Care for Uncomplicated Pregnancies, Clinical Guideline CG62.* London: NICE [https://www.nice.org.uk/guidance/cg62].

National Institute for Health and Clinical Excellence (NICE) (2012) *Preventing Type 2 Diabetes: Risk identification and interventions for individuals at high risk*, Public Health Guidline PH38. London: NICE [https://www.nice.org.uk/guidance/ph38].

National Institute for Health and Clinical Excellence (NICE) (2015) *Diabetes in Pregnancy: Management from preconception to the postnatal period*, NICE Guideline NG3. London: NICE [https://www.nice.org.uk/guidance/ng3].

Nielsen, L.R., Pedersen-Bjergaard, U., Thorsteinsson, B., Johansen, M., Damm, P. and Mathiesen, E.R. (2008) Hypoglycemia in pregnant women with type 1 diabetes: predictors and role of metabolic control. *Diabetes Care*, 31(1): 9–14.

O'Sullivan, J., Gellis, S., Dandrow, R. and Tenney, B. (1966) The potential diabetic and her treatment in pregnancy. *Obstetrics and Gynaecology*, 27 (5): 683–9.

Royal College of Obstetricians and Gynaecologists (RCOG) (2011) Diabetes and treatment of gestational diabetes, *Scientific Advisory Committee Opinion Paper 23*, January. London: RCOG.

Russell, C., Dodds, L., Armson, B.A., Kephart, G. and Joseph, K.S. (2008) Diabetes mellitus following gestational diabetes: role of subsequent pregnancy, *BJOG: An International Journal of Obstetrics and Gynaecology*, 115 (2): 253–60.

Sherridan, A. (2013) Circle of defence and line of authority: breastfeeding peer counsellors' reflections on their support role in a northern town, *MIDIRS Midwifery Digest*, 23 (1): 95–100.

Spyer, G. (2008) Pregnancy in MODY, in *Diabetes in Pregnancy: The scientific basis for clinical practice*. Educational launch of the NICE guideline 'Diabetes in Pregnancy', 7–8 April 2008, RCOG, London.

Stenhouse, E., Letherby, G. and Stephen, N. (2013) Women with pre-existing diabetes and their experiences of maternity care services, *Midwifery*, 29 (2): 148–53.

Temple, R. (2008) Severe hypoglycaemia and hyperglycaemia in pregnancy, in *Diabetes in Pregnancy: The scientific basis for clinical practice*. Educational launch of the NICE guideline 'Diabetes in Pregnancy', 7–8 April 2008, RCOG, London.

Tyer-Viola, L.A. and Lopez, R.P. (2014) Pregnancy with chronic illness, *Journal of Obstetric, Gynecologic and Neonatal Nursing*, 43 (1): 25–37.

Vaxillaire, M. and Froguel, P. (2006) Genetic basis of maturity-onset diabetes of the young, *Endocrinology and Metabolism Clinics of North America*, 35 (2): 371–84.

World Health Organization (WHO) (1996) *Care in Normal Birth: A practical guide*. Geneva: WHO.

World Health Organization (WHO) (1999) *Definition, Diagnosis and Classification of Diabetes Mellitus and its Complications*. Geneva: WHO.

World Health Organization (WHO) (2011) *Use of Glycated Haemoglobin (HbA1C) in the Diagnosis of Diabetes Mellitus*. Geneva: WHO.

World Health Organization (WHO) (2013) *Diagnostic Criteria and Classification of Hyperglycaemia when First Detected in Pregnancy*. Geneva: WHO.

Yim, I.S., Glynn, L.M., Dunkel-Schetter, C., Hobel, C.J., Chicz-Demet, A. and Sandman, C.A. (2009) Risk of postpartum depressive symptoms with elevated corticotrophin hormone in human pregnancy, *Archives of General Psychiatry*, 66 (2): 162–9.

Yorkshire and Humber Public Health Observatory (2010) *Diabetes Prevalence Model (APHO)* [http://www.yhpho.org.uk/resource/view.aspx?RID=81090; accessed 2 June 2014].

Index

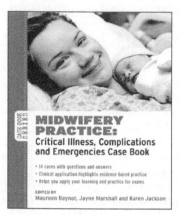

MIDWIFERY PRACTICE
Critical Illness, Complications and
Emergencies Case Book

Maureen Raynor, Jayne Marshall and
Karen Jackson

9780335242733 (Paperback)
May 2012

eBook also available

Part of a case book series, this book contains 14 common pregnancy and
childbirth emergency scenarios to help prepare student midwives for life in
practice. Each case explores and explains the pathology, pharmacology and
care principles, and uses test questions and answers to help assess learning.

Key features:

- Covers the principles, pathology and skills involved in a range of
  birthing scenarios
- Each chapter includes Q&A's, further resources, pre-requisite
  learning, summaries, boxes and learning tools in order to track and
  further learning
- The practical cases will help you link theory to practice

www.openup.co.uk

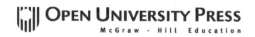 **OPEN UNIVERSITY PRESS**
M c G r a w - H i l l   E d u c a t i o n